Me

Syed Fazl-e-Haider

Medical Palmistry in Practice

A Palmistry Guide to Diagnosis of Diseases

VDM Verlag Dr. Müller

Impressum/Imprint (nur für Deutschland/ only for Germany)

Bibliografische Information der Deutschen Nationalbibliothek: Die Deutsche Nationalbibliothek verzeichnet diese Publikation in der Deutschen Nationalbibliografie; detaillierte bibliografische Daten sind im Internet über http://dnb.d-nb.de abrufbar.

Alle in diesem Buch genannten Marken und Produktnamen unterliegen warenzeichen-, marken- oder patentrechtlichem Schutz bzw. sind Warenzeichen oder eingetragene Warenzeichen der jeweiligen Inhaber. Die Wiedergabe von Marken, Produktnamen, Gebrauchsnamen, Handelsnamen, Warenbezeichnungen u.s.w. in diesem Werk berechtigt auch ohne besondere Kennzeichnung nicht zu der Annahme, dass solche Namen im Sinne der Warenzeichen- und Markenschutzgesetzgebung als frei zu betrachten wären und daher von jedermann benutzt werden dürften.

Coverbild: www.ingimage.com

Verlag: VDM Verlag Dr. Müller GmbH & Co. KG
Dudweiler Landstr. 99, 66123 Saarbrücken, Deutschland
Telefon +49 681 9100-698, Telefax +49 681 9100-988
Email: info@vdm-verlag.de

Herstellung in Deutschland:
Schaltungsdienst Lange o.H.G., Berlin
Books on Demand GmbH, Norderstedt
Reha GmbH, Saarbrücken
Amazon Distribution GmbH, Leipzig
ISBN: 978-3-639-26619-1

Imprint (only for USA, GB)

Bibliographic information published by the Deutsche Nationalbibliothek: The Deutsche Nationalbibliothek lists this publication in the Deutsche Nationalbibliografie; detailed bibliographic data are available in the Internet at http://dnb.d-nb.de.

Any brand names and product names mentioned in this book are subject to trademark, brand or patent protection and are trademarks or registered trademarks of their respective holders. The use of brand names, product names, common names, trade names, product descriptions etc. even without a particular marking in this works is in no way to be construed to mean that such names may be regarded as unrestricted in respect of trademark and brand protection legislation and could thus be used by anyone.

Cover image: www.ingimage.com

Publisher: VDM Verlag Dr. Müller GmbH & Co. KG
Dudweiler Landstr. 99, 66123 Saarbrücken, Germany
Phone +49 681 9100-698, Fax +49 681 9100-988
Email: info@vdm-publishing.com

Printed in the U.S.A.
Printed in the U.K. by (see last page)
ISBN: 978-3-639-26619-1

Medical Palmistry in Practice

A Palmistry Guide to Diagnosis of Diseases

BY

Syed Fazl-e-Haider

__Contents__

Preface

__PART - I__

PART - II

MEDICAL CHIROGNOMY

PART III

MEDICAL CHIROMANCY

PART IV

PALMISTIC DATA FOR VARIOUS DISORDERS

Preface

It was during my school-going days that I took interest in Palmistry. I studied a number of books, as my interest developed to understand the mysteries, which the lines and signs of hand unfold. What inspired me the most in palmistry were the scientific aspects of hand-reading. Then I began to read hands on scientific lines. I discarded all occultism, skepticism and traditionalism in hand-analysis and directed my efforts to find empirical evidences through research and practical work in the field of medical Palmistry. I personally met with many patients and analyzed their hands. Being a journalist by profession, I got the opportunities to review the hands of people from different walks of life. I also wrote columns on Palmistry in newspapers for a long time.

'Medical Palmistry in Practice' is a deviation from the traditional perception of hand-analysis to a scientific perception of immense diagnostic value in Medicine. There are two schools of thought, which deliver judgment on the study of palmistry- 1) Traditional school of thought, and 2) Modern/Scientific school of thought. The traditional school of thought considers Palmistry as an art of fortune-telling and the Palmist a fortune-teller. I want to make it clear that there is nothing like fortune-telling in this book.

Modern/Scientific school of thought considers Palmistry a science related to the human psychology and the Palmist a hand-analyst analyzing different hand-features on scientific lines. The book has been written with an aim to draw the attention of medical doctors toward the research studies undertaken and ongoing scientific research in the field of medical Palmistry and resultantly benefit from the empirical evidences that have come out of these studies. In Europe, America, India and many other countries, Palmistry has emerged as a science from the medical point of view equally helpful both for doctors and patients alike in diagnosing the diseases.

When you go to a doctor for the treatment of some disease you are ill with, the doctor first proceeds to the diagnosis of the aliment through medical checkup carried out by examination of different organs of your body in order to find the symptoms disclosing the specific disease. Sometimes, he examines your heart-beat or checks your blood pressure. Often he observes the fingernails and tries to note the texture, shape and different signs formed on the nails. This medical checkup leads the doctor to the diagnosis of the disease you are suffering from.

The medical palmistry in fact, is the field of study of different signs and indications found in the hand by which common diseases of human body can be diagnosed. It is a medical fact that nerves connected from brain to hand are highly developed and our hand contains more nerves than any other portion of the body.

Brain is considered to be the powerhouse of our body, which stores all powers vital to a normal functioning of systems of our body (specifying the health of the entire body) like power of decision, power of survival, power of revival, power of concentration, power of confrontation, will power and so on.

As power-house of the body, brain generates electricity in the form of nerve-impulses, which pass through wires or nerves traversing the whole human body. These nerves form a highly complicated net-work along with another network of capillaries (microscopic blood vessels) spreading over in the entire human body.

In view of highly developed and largely connected nerves from brain to hand, our hand is considered to be the recorder of brain actions, mental pursuits and intellectual activities. Being power-house of the body, action of brain affects our entire body and as recorder of brain's actions, hand records these effects in the form of Palmistic markings.

Brain functions normally in a normal person. The function of the brain is however, affected by a physical or psychological disorder. Action of brain affects entire body. Likewise, any disorder in the physiology of the body affects the brain first, and it functions abnormally. This abnormality appears as Palmistic sign in the hand.

Modern/Scientific school of thought has based its judgement on empirical evidences obtained from sampling and different research methodologies. This school considers Palmistry a science related to human Psychology. It is a study of Mind. The palm of a person has a close and direct relation with his brain. According to the Scientific school, the optimistic thinking creates straight lines on palm whereas pessimistic thinking creates many lines and broken lines on palm.

In Europe and America, thousands of scientific studies have been undertaken on the subjects like 'hand & fertility', 'hand & personality, 'hand & Health', 'hand & psychology' and so on. Empirical evidences have also been found that certain skin ridges, palmar patterns, markings on nails and line formations are more common in particular syndromes or diseases. For example, The Simian Line has been found to be more common in genetic disorders such as Down's syndrome.

This can very rightly be concluded," normal action of brain specifies a normal body with normal functioning of its systems. It is however, undeniable fact that nobody is perfect and perfectly normal. How can we distinguish between a normal and an abnormal thing? " *Anything beyond normal is abnormal.,"* is the logical principle applied in this book for predicting an abnormality or disease of the body through analysis of hand. It is also a fact that there are no accepted set of rules for declaring a thing normal. A thing or point may be normal for one, but same may be abnormal for the other. Everybody has his own definition or criteria for a thing or action to be normal. This rule has just been given to create a format, as accepted by most of the authorities on Palmistry for the hand-analyst.

Before applying this simple but logical rule to a person's hand, a criterion for normal hand and the lines of hand within the parameters of medical palmistry has been given in the book. It is, however, necessary to mention that knowledge being provided by me on medical palmistry is limited and by no means complete but interesting and equally important both for general readers and experts. It is mainly purported to draw attention of medical doctors, researchers and experts toward field of medical palmistry opening doors to a thorough and well-organized research in the field.

I want to clarify that I am not a Palmist or doctor by profession. Whatever work I did in this regard is mainly aimed at opening new vistas or avenues for research in the field of medical hand-analysis. The men of the field including doctors, psychiatrists, sociologists and criminologists should come forward, undertake new studies and apply this science for diagnosis of diseases and deviate behaviors in the society for the benefit of all.

Syed Fazl-e-Haider,

The Author

Acknowledgment

I cannot forget the help of my friends in undertaking research studies. I would like to mention here the name of Amanullah Kakar, one of my best friends, who facilitated my research studies. He was the student Social Work Department of the University of Balochistan during 2001. He collected for me the prints of the hands of Psycho patients, drug addicts and the convicts (Jailbirds) whom he met during his survey work as a student of Social Work.

I would like to remember here my cousin Dr. Fauzia Hashmi, who provided me the literature on physiology and anatomy and also helped me on medical side of the research.

I would specially mention here the name of my friend Asad Shah, who provided me all technical help in every stage of book compilation. I would also name Syed Usman Ali, Abdul Rehman, Hasan Panizai, Tariq Hasmi and Abu Bakar, as they all supported me in my research work.

Dedicated to

I dedicate this book to my Parents- My father, Syed Nazir Ali Shah and my mother Shamima Khatoon, who ever prayed for my success.

PART - I

Chap: No. 1

Hand & Brain

1) Anatomy of Hand

    i) Nerves of the hand

    ii) Arteries of the hand

    iii) Blood Capillaries in the Hand

2- Some Facts about 'Brain '

    i) Localization of function

    ii) Brain controls & guides behavior

    iii) Eye-hand coordination in split brain

CHAP: NO. 1

Hand & Brain

1. Anatomy of the hand

The anatomy of the hand is complex and fascinating. Its integrity is absolutely essential for our everyday functional living. Medical science recognizes that the nerves connected from brain to hand are larger in number than any other part of the human body. For this reason the hand is considered as the mirror of brain. The nerves, which connect the brain with the hands, belong to the "Brachial plexus."

The "Brachial Plexus" is the cluster of nerves which is formed by the interlacing of interior branches of the last cervical pairs and the first dorsal. It is further divided into median nerve and cubical nerve. "Touch Corpuscles" are those small bodies, which are connected with the cutaneous nerves of the palm ending in a nervous filament. The nerves of the touch communicate with the touch corpuscles, which render the sense of more acute.

The skin of the dorsum of the hand is thin and pliable. It is attached to the hand's skeleton only by loose areolar tissue, where lymphatics and veins course. The skin of the palmar surface of the hand is unique, with characteristics for special function. The palmar skin is thick and glabrous and not as pliable as the dorsal skin. It is strongly attached to the underlying fascia by numerous vertical fibers. These features enhance the skin stability for proper grasping function.

The skin is most firmly anchored to the deep structures at the palmar creases; this is of clinical importance when planning surgical incisions to minimize skin contractures. In contrast to the dorsal skin, the blood supply to the palmar skin is through numerous small vertical branches from the common digital vessels. Therefore, the elevation of palmar skin flaps is limited. Finally, the skin of the palmar surface of the hand contains a high concentration of sensory nerve organs essential to the hand's normal function.

The nails are specialized skin appendages derived from the epidermis. The nail bed has a germinal matrix, sterile matrix and hyponychium. Ninety percent of the nail plate is produced by the germinal matrix, which approximately corresponds to the lunula (pale semicircle in proximal nail bed). This germinal matrix starts proximally at the base of the distal phalanx just distal to the insertion of the extensor tendon. The nail matrix distal to the lunula is called the sterile matrix; it is very vascular, which accounts for the pink color. The sterile matrix produces 10% of nail plate volume and adds squamous components, which make the nail stronger and adherent to the nail bed. The hyponychium is the distal part of the nail bed; its abundance of immune cells and adherence to the distal nail plate help resist nail infection.

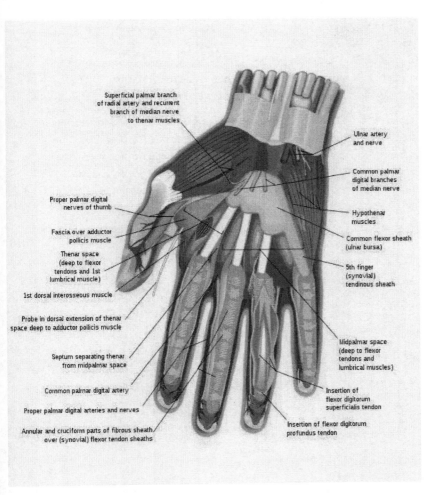

Fig. 1.1   **Anatomy of Hand**

The anatomy of the hand shows that it contains several nerves, arteries, veins and capillaries.

A) Nerves of the hand

The hand is innervated by three nerves: the median, ulnar and radial nerves. Each has both sensory and motor components. Variations from the classic nerve distribution are so common that they are the rule rather than the exception. The skin of the forearm is innervated medially by the medial antebrachial cutaneous nerve and laterally by the lateral antebrachial cutaneous nerve.

The median nerve is responsible for innervating the muscles involved in the fine precision and pinch function of the hand. The ulnar nerve is responsible for innervating the muscles involved in the power grasping function of the hand. The radial nerve is responsible for innervating the wrist extensors, which control the position of the hand and stabilizes the fixed unit. The skin of the hand is supplied by the spinal nerves through the median and the ulnar nerves.

The hand actually contains three main nerves and their countless branches:

1. Ulnar nerve

2. Median nerve

3. Radial nerve

1. **Ulnar Nerve**

It is the main nerve of the hand, which enters the palm and divides into two branches:

a) *SUPERFICIAL TERMINAL BRANCH:*

This supplies one and half fingers.

b) *DEEP TERMINAL BRANCH:*

This supplies muscles and wrist joint.

Ulnar nerve originates at the medial cord of the brachial plexus. Motor branches innervate the flexor carpi ulnaris and flexor digitorum profundus muscles to the ring and small fingers. Proximal to the wrist, the palmar cutaneous branch provides sensation at the hypothenar eminence. The dorsal branch, which branches from the main trunk at the distal forearm, provides sensation to the ulnar portion of the dorsum of the hand and small finger, and part of the ring finger. At the hand, the superficial branch forms the digital nerves, which provide sensation at the small finger and ulnar aspect of the ring finger.

The deep motor branch passes through the Guyon canal in company with the ulnar artery. It innervates the hypothenar muscles (abductor digiti minimi, opponens digiti minimi, flexor digiti minimi, and palmaris brevis), all interossei, the 2 ulnar lumbricals, the adductor pollicis, and the deep head of the flexor pollicis brevis.

2.   Median Nerve

It is an important nerve, which controls the movement of the thumb. The median nerve enters the palm and divides into lateral and medial branches:

a) The lateral branch divides into 3-digital branches for lateral one and half digits including the thumb.

b) The medial branch divides into two digital branches for second and third clefts.

Median nerve originates from the lateral and medial cords of the brachial plexus. In the forearm, the motor branches supply the pronator teres, flexor carpi radialis, palmaris longus, and flexor digitorum superficialis muscles. The anterior interosseus branch innervates the flexor pollicis longus, flexor digitorum profundus (index and long finger), and pronator quadratus muscles.

Proximal to the wrist, the palmar cutaneous branch provides sensation at the thenar eminence. As the median nerve passes through the carpal tunnel, the recurrent motor branch innervates the thenar muscles (abductor pollicis brevis, opponens pollicis, and superficial head of flexor pollicis brevis).7 It also innervates the index and long finger lumbrical muscles. Sensory digital branches provide sensation to the thumb, index, long, and radial side of the ring finger.

3.   Radial Nerve

This nerve is distributed to the proximal parts of the dorsal surfaces of the thumb, the index finger and the lateral half of the middle finger.

Radial nerve originates from the posterior cord of the brachial plexus. At the elbow, motor branches innervate the brachioradialis and extensor carpi radialis longus muscles. At the proximal forearm, the radial nerve divides into the superficial and deep branches. The deep posterior interosseous branch innervates all the muscles in the extensor compartment: supinator, extensor carpi radialis brevis, extensor digitorum communis, extensor digiti minimi, extensor carpi ulnaris, extensor indicis proprius, extensor pollicis longus, extensor pollicis brevis, and abductor pollicis longus. The superficial branch provides sensation at the radial aspect of the dorsum of the hand, the dorsum of the thumb, and the dorsum of the index, long, and radial half of the ring finger proximal to the distal interphalangeal joints.

B) Arteries of the hand

The main arteries and their branches of the hand are as follows:

1. Ulnar artery

2. Radial artery

When these two arteries unite, they form superficial and deep palmer arches.

1. Ulnar Artery

After entering the palm it ends by dividing into two branches, namely:

a) *Superficial palmer branch,* which is the main continuation of the artery.

b) *Deep palmer branch,* which arises from in front of the flexor rectinaculum immediately beyond the pisiform bone. These two branches of ulnar artery form the superficial and deep palmer arches.

2. Radial Artery

After entering the palm, it runs medially and divides into two branches namely,

a) *The radial indices branch,* which supplies blood to the radial side of the index finger.

b) *Princeps pollics branch,* which supplies blood to the thumb.

C) Blood Capillaries in the Hand

The microscopic blood vessels formed by the division and re-division of blood arteries and veins are called as blood capillaries. There is a network of blood capillaries along with the lines of the hand. The blood circulates through these capillaries to bathe the living cells and tissues of the hand. Our body has a closed type of blood circulatory system in which the blood passes through the blood vessel to maintain normal condition.

2- Some Facts about 'Brain '

i) Localization of function

With the exception of brain, in any organ of the human body, one part of the organ performs the same function as any other part. For instance, any part of kidney, lung or liver performs much the same function as the other part does. Therefore, in case of serious disorder, quite a large affected fraction of the organ can be destroyed without fatally affecting the particular function of the whole organ. This is a well-known fact that a man can survive and lead a normal physical life with one kidney (in the absence of other kidney), as one kidney performs the same function of urine formation as the pair of kidneys does.

It is an established fact that the structure and function of brain is highly complicated. Different parts of brain perform different functions. This localization of function is the single most important difference between the brain and rest of the human body. On account of this localization of function, a small focal lesion in brain can produce a severe but selective deficit in a single function.

ii) Brain controls & guides behavior

Psychological research confirms that the brain not only controls and guides behavior but is also responsive. It is a dynamic system responsive to environmental stimulation and capable of self-modification.

The brain is organized in three integrated layers: the brain stem and cerebellum, the limbic system and the cerebral cortex. The brain stem and cerebellum control survival functions and locomotion, the limbic system maintains balance in motivation and emotion, and the cerebral cortex controls complex mental activity.

The cerebral cortex is responsible for consciousness. It is divided into two hemispheres connected by the corpus callosum. While the hemispheres are physically symmetrical, their processing styles are not. The Language, analytical thinking and positive emotions are regulated by the left hemisphere, while the right hemisphere controls spatial interpretations, facial recognition and negative emotions. Although severing the corpus callosum can create dual consciousness, the brain is designed to function as an integrated whole.

iii) Eye-hand coordination in split brain

The research study on ' Eye-hand coordination in split brain subjects' indicates that when a split-brain patient uses the left hand to find a match to an object appearing in the left visual field, eye-hand coordination is normal, because both are registered in the right hemisphere. But when asked to use the right hand to match an object seen in the left visual field, the patient cannot perform the task and mismatches a pear with a cup.

This is because of the fact that sensations from the right hand go to the left hemisphere, and there is no longer a connection between the two hemispheres.

Besides the nervous disorders, most diseases of the brain have their counterparts in other organs of the body. So diseases with systemic counterparts badly affect the function of brain producing different manifestations, which are recorded by hand (as recorder of brain's actions) in the form of different signs on palm.

In this way, not only the diseases of brain but diseases of rest of the body can be diagnosed through a careful scrutiny of hand and palmistic markings, and on the basis of palmistic data collected, the medical palmist can wonderfully predict the diseases of a subject, he may prone. For centuries, Medicine has recognized the link between Palmistry and good health. Plato, Anaxagoras and Galen have emphasized in their writings the importance of the hand in the study of human beings.

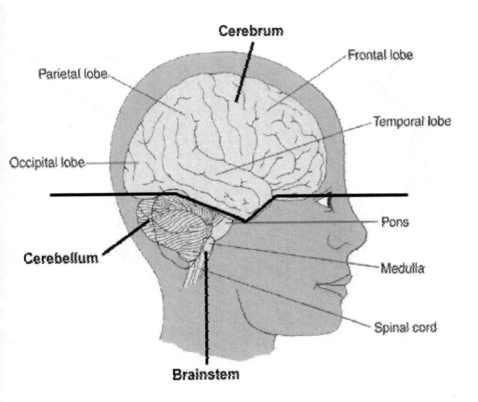

Fig. 1.2   Human Brain

CHAP. NO. 2

Formation of Lines

i) Neural activity

ii) Thinking, a higher-order mental process

iii) Neurotransmission

CHAP. NO.2

Formation of Lines

The anatomy of hand shows that the hand contains more nerves than any part of the body. It also denotes that hand contains countless blood vessels- veins, arteries and capillaries, which are originally, connected with the vital organ of body- the heart. The blood circulation or transportation in the body is affected by mental disorder or some psycho-physical disorder. Therefore it can rightly be concluded:

"The lines of the hands are formed due to mental processes- thinking and production of ideas- and change due to change in our thinking and ideas". If changes occur due to some disease affecting the function of brain, then the lines or signs which appear on the palm, nails or any portion of the hand will reveal the specific disease, the subject is suffering from or may prone.

The nerves of the body transmit and receive messages from the brain through the electrical impulses transmitting through the nerves. Now question is that how are these impulses produced and how they cause formation or alteration of lines on the palm?

i) Neural activity

Neural activity is the biological medium in which behavior, thinking and emotion all occur. Changes in nervous system activity lead to the changes in how people behave, think and feel.

ii) Thinking, a higher-order mental process

Thinking is a higher-order mental process that goes beyond the information given by sensory processing. Psychologists believe that 'Thinking' is a complex mental process of forming a new representation by transforming available information.

That information involves the interaction of many mental activities, such as inferring, abstracting, reasoning, imagining, judging, problem solving, and, at times, creativity. Thinking relies on a variety of mental structures.

These structures include concepts, schemes, scripts and visual imagery. Taking together, these mental structures form the basis how we think so efficiently.

iii) Neurotransmission

The nervous system uses electrochemical signals to process and transmit information. A single neuron's electrical activity changes when electrically charged particles called ions flow through the membrane that separates the cell's inside from the outside environment. The biochemical substances that stimulate other neurons are called as neurotransmitters. More than 60 different chemical substances are known or suspected to function as neurotransmitters in brain. The gap between the two neurons is called synapse.

The process by which the information is relayed from one neuron to another across the synaptic gap is called synaptic transmission. All nervous system activity depends on synaptic transmission.

In fact, our thoughts, ideas and mental processes are responsible for producing the nerve-impulses. As stated before, nerves connected from brain to hand are larger in number and hand is considered as the mirror of brain, therefore our thoughts, ideas and other mental processes appear on palm in the form of lines and different signs.

According to the scientific school of Palmistry, the current of life enters the human body through Index finger (First Finger). It marks the Line of Heart on the palm and then Line of Head and finally the Line of Life. After reaching the wrist on its return journey, it makes Line of Sun, Line of Saturn and Line of Mercury.

Fingers connect the human body with the outside world. They work as a transmitter to spread the electrical currents or thoughts of our mind generated in the brain to the environment. In the same way fingers also work as a receiver of electrical currents or thoughts different people receive from the environment and carry it to the brain. These electrical currents or thoughts help in the formation and changing of line.

CHAP. NO. 3

What Is Medical Palmistry?

i) Views of Modern researchers

ii) Basis of Medical Palmistry

iii) Branches of Medical Palmistry

iv) Importance of 'Dermatoglyphics'

CHAP. NO. 3

What Is Medical Palmistry?

The branch of palmistry, which deals with the diagnosis of diseases from palm, nails and lines of the hands, is called medical palmistry. For centuries now, Medicine has recognized the link between Palmistry and good health. Plato stressed the importance of the hand in the study of human beings, Aristotle furthered this application and Hippocrates practiced this art on all his patients.

1) Views of Modern Researchers

Modern medical researchers have also confirmed the link between Palmistry and good health. Dr Satish Tadwalkar, a Medical Palmist in India said, "Your palm could indicate the early warning symptoms to your health and serve as a guide for all your physical and mental ailments."

William Benham, the author of 'The Laws of Scientific Hand Reading' said:-

"No help was found from professionals, for nearly all proved to be ignorant, unlettered, and trying solely to gain money, without any effort in the direction of scientific investigation. During most of this time the word palmistry was so buried under a mass of public disapproval, that a self respecting person dared not say that he was even interested in it. Fully persuaded that it had a scientific foundation, I set about to discover it."

During his practice, Prof. Daya Nand, the founder of institute of Palmistry in India, discovered certain facts about lines of hand and shape of hand, which encouraged him to study further deeper the science of palmistry.

According to Prof. Daya Nand, palmistry is a study of unconscious mind, which has close relation with our brain and thinking power. He believes that a palmist is like a physician. The physician heals the body and good palmist heals mind through remedies. Remedies help to change inauspicious to auspicious.

2) Basis of Medical Palmistry

The medical palmistry is based upon a suggested theory of lines formation by which we come to know that the development of lines is due to mental processes and activities, which appear as lines or signs on the palm of our hands. A careful analysis of these lines or signs leads us to the diagnosis of many diseases or health problems, a person could face in life.

According to the practitioners of medical palmistry, "As our thought and ideas change with time, so the lines of the hand appear, disappear and change with our changing ideas."

3) Branches of Medical Palmistry

For an effective study, the field of medical palmistry has been divided into three branches:

I.   Medical Chirognomy

This is the branch of medical palmistry in which hereditary traits, nature, temperament and other physical and Psychological complications of a subject are predicted through a careful analysis of shapes of hands and fingers.

II.   Medical Chiromancy

This is branch of medical palmistry in which diseases of the body are diagnosed through an analysis of lines of the hand and other signs and markings, which appear on the palm.

Chirognomically, a careful analysis of shape of hand and fingers and also color of skin of a person's hand reveals his proclivities, trends, hereditary traits, nature and his temperament which help the medical palmist in predicting physical aliments and psychic disorders, the person may prone. However, for making such prediction proficiency in the subject (gained through a thorough research) is a pre-requisite. Therefore a medical palmist must be extremely cautious while predicting a disease.

III. Palmar Dermatoglyphics

Palmar Dermatoglyphs is the branch of medical palmistry which deals with the study of skin ridges in the hands. All studies of the dermal ridge arrangements including genetics and anthropology are classified under the term 'dermatoglyphics'.

4) Importance of 'Dermatoglyphics'

In this book, the Dermatoglyphics is not the topic of discussion. However, some information on the subject is given for the readers' interest.

The word dermatoglyphics comes from two Greek words- *derma* means skin, while *glyph* means carve- and refers to the friction ridge formations which appear on the palms of the hands. The hair does not grow from this area. The ridging formations serve well to enhance contact, an area of multiple nerve endings (Dermal Papillae).

The ridge formations of the skin of an individual begin to appear during the third and fourth month of fetal development. After death, decomposition of the skin is last to occur in the area of the dermatoglyphic configurations.

Historically, the ridges of the hands have been attracting the medical researches and palmists of different countries for centuries. But the first attempt to systematically categorized fingerprint patterns is found in the work of Purkinje who wrote initial paper in 1880. He used a nine pattern classification.

The studies exploring the hereditary aspects of fingerprints, investigating comparisons of siblings, twins and genetically unrelated individuals and concordance of papillary ridge patterns among relatives have also been undertaken. This aroused the interest of anthropologists in dermatoglyphics.

Dermal palmer ridges are highly useful in biological studies. Scientific studies regarding the methodology, inheritance and racial variation of palmer and planter papillary ridge patterns as well as fingerprints have been undertaken in the world.

The importance of ridge patterns has been recognized by different schools of palmistry. The modern investigators of Palmistry have expressed keen interest in the dermal ridges. The research studies have found major psychological connections of fingerprints and individual subjects. For example, the whorl pattern has commonly been found on the prints of certain types of criminals.

By the early 1980's, DNA testing had replaced the dermatoglyphic test as the standard in twin studies, issues of paternity, and chromosome disorder research. The Genome Project, a "big science" project that intends to fully map human DNA within the next several years, has gobbled up the funding that used to sustain dermatoglyphic research.

Terry Reed, who has been teaching dermatoglyphics at the University of Indiana Department of Medical Genetics, concludes that "Until the major genetic disorders have been mapped and sequenced, it will likely be several years before a shift occurs towards the study of normal morphological traits, such as dermatoglyphics...When this happens, the results may prove to be quite fascinating."

The several possible applications of dermatoglyphics seem quite promising.

Some important applications are:

- Dermatoglyphics may be applied as primary means of assessing complex genetic traits

- Because fingerprints and line formations form during vital stages of fetal development, dermatoglyphic studies are in a unique position to evaluate the effect of toxins on the intrauterine environment (over 20% of all pregnancies never come to term).

- Dermatoglyphics are still useful for the evaluation of children with suspected genetic disorders and diseases with long latency, slow progression, and late onset.

CHAP. NO. 4

Scope of Medical Palmistry

i) Benefits & Applications of Medical Palmistry

ii) Medical Palmistry as study of Human psychology

iii) Palmistry- A Science Related to Brain & Thinking Power

CHAP. NO. 4

Scope of Medical Palmistry

Medical palmistry is in fact the branch of medical science with a great and wider scope in Medicine. It can be employed in the prediction of many diseases like jaundice, anemia, tuberculosis, brain tumor, heart diseases, lungs diseases, and psychic disease and so on. A careful analysis of hand may lead to the diagnosis of the symptoms and indications resulting in cancer or AIDS.

Medical palmistry is the science of great significance due to its vast applications and merits. However, a need is still felt to undertake more research to aware the people of the importance of this useful science. Medical Palmistry not only helps diagnosing diseases but it also helps one to know about the patient's temperament, his/her constitution, and the subconscious mind. Besides, some factors such as love, libido, and the emotions that are beyond the pale of empirical sciences, can easily be recognized by the knowledge of Palmistry, which plays the role of computers for the body.

i) Benefits & Applications of Medical Palmistry

Some authorities have enumerated the following important benefits and applications of Medical Palmistry:

1) It provides an early warning for forthcoming diseases, and one can prevent them early.

2) It provides information about hidden diseases, which remain, undiagnosed or misdiagnosed by doctors.

3) It helps in the prognosis of diseases where doctors are unsure about it.

4) Psychological ailments can be easily recognized by the study of the palm.

5) Palmistry has a major role in prevention of diseases. With its help and knowledge, a doctor can easily recognize the weakness of the system and

advise the patient all relevant nutritional changes to prevent the disease from becoming severe.

Modern researchers believe that:

I) Medical Palmistry is related to Human Psychology.

II) Medical Palmistry is a science related to Human brain and thinking power.

ii) Medical Palmistry- A Study of Human Psychology

Modern researchers believe that Medical palmistry is related to human psychology. Psychology is the scientific study of the behavior of individuals and their mental processes.

Observable behaviors such as speaking, running or taking a rest can be directly observed, but an individual's mental processes cannot. Many human activities are really private and internal events: reasoning, creating and dreaming. Many psychologists believe that such mental processes, though not directly observable, represent the most important subject of psychology inquiry. This inquiry can best be conducted through medical Palmistry.

Medical Palmistry is a study of unconscious mind. When psychology first emerged as distinctive science from philosophy and other sciences in the late 1800s, it became the 'science of mind'; the mind's major work consisted of producing consciousness.

The way psychology conceptualizes consciousness has been influenced by an ongoing debate about how mind and brain are related. Materialistic theories argue that brain and mind are the same.

With the emergence of neuroscience, the biologically oriented psychologists supported the position that the mind and brain were identical. After all, the brain has vast resources; we cannot begin to comprehend- approximately 100 billion neurons, each with thousands of individual and collective interconnections, and degrees of firing strength. Surely, the human brain is capable of much more than we imagined, including the universe of imagination we think of as mind.

In this materialistic view, the brain is sort of super machine and its primary product is mind. From this perspective, the mind is what the brain does, and only biological-materialistic explanations are required to understand their equivalence. In this view, any creature with a brain, therefore, also has a mind, whether it is human being, a lion, computer or a robot.

Roger Sperry and Michael Gazzaniga challenged this materialistic theory during 1970s, and they presented the emergent-interaction theory of mind-brain relationship.

The emergent-interaction theory proposes that while brain activities create mental states, they are not the same things, and brain and mind interact and influence each other.

Today, the Psychologists are of the considered view that it is not possible, either scientifically or logically, to prove or disprove the existence of mind. The mind is by definition something each person experiences subjectively. Ultimately, then accepting the existence of one's own mind remains a matter of faith. However, the mental function of greatest interest to psychologists is consciousness.

A basic question that psychology asks is this: What is the nature of human nature? The psychologists answer this question by looking at processes that occur within individuals as well as within the physical and social environment.

The medical palmistry can, in fact answer this basic question of the psychology by revealing the nature of human nature through a careful analysis of certain hand-features, lines and signs on the palm.

iii) Palmistry- A Science Related to Brain & Thinking Power

The brain is a complex organ whose interrelated elements are held in delicate balance. Subtle alterations in the brain's tissue or in its chemical messengers (neurotransmitters) can have significant effects. Genetic factors, brain injury and infection are a few of the causes of these alterations.

Technological advances in brain scanning techniques have enabled biologically oriented researchers to discover links between psychological disorders and specific brain abnormalities. For example, extreme violence has been linked to brain tumors located in an area of the brain associated with aggressive behavior. Today researchers increasingly view psychopathology as the product of a complex interaction between a number of biological and psychological factors.

Psychologists have found evidence that the negative emotional states such as depression, anxiety, and hostility can affect physical conditions such as coronary disease, asthma, headache, gastric ulcers and arthritis. The chronic negative emotional states tend to produce pathogenic (disease-causing) changes in the body, unhealthy behavior patterns and poor personal relationships.

The body's two communication systems are the nervous system and the endocrine system. The nervous system composed of billions of neurons is further subdivided into central nervous system (CNS) and the peripheral nervous system (PNS). The nerve cell or neuron receives processes and relays information to other cells, glands and muscles. Sensory neurons send messages toward the CNS; motor neurons channel messages from the CNS; and interneurons relay information between neurons. Glia bind neurons together.

When a neuron fires, information is relayed from the dendrites, through the soma, and through the axon to the terminal buttons. Neurotransmitters are released into the synaptic gap, where they may be taken up by the receiving neuron.

Endocrine communication not only sustains our slow and continuous bodily processes, but also helps us to respond in crises. Hormones are secreted into the bloodstream by endocrine glands.

Hormones are involved in a wide array of bodily functions and behaviors. They influence body growth, sexual development, arousal, mood and metabolism. Hypothalamus is the brain center in charge of the endocrine.

Good health means a perfect balance between the body, mind and soul. This can be gauged by the knowledge of Medical Palmistry. Hippocrates, the Father of Medicine, Aristotle, the founder of psychology, and Dr Charles Bell, the Father of Modern Neurology, all studied the human hand as a diagnostic aid. Today, Medical Palmistry is not an occult science. It is a science of diagnosing symptoms of diseases in the hand.

Our hands indicate the symptoms of the diseases before the infection takes place. Therefore with the help of medical palmistry, the subject can be made aware of the coming health problems; he may suffer, by just observing the signs or indication of that specific disease in the hand. Medical palmistry is a useful science, which helps in knowing the psychology, mentality and the intellectual trend of a subject. It predicts about his nature, mental proclivities, physical health and his inherent capabilities.

Medical science has recognized that only through the analysis of nails, several diseases can be predicted. The experts are of the opinion that the nail of index finger is related to the liver, the second finger-nail to the skeleton, the third finger-nail to the Cardio-renal system, the fourth to the nervous system and the nail of thumb is related to the cerebral system.

I am certain, if a research is made in this field on scientific grounds, medical palmistry would be very helpful in the diagnosis of diseases.

CHAP. NO. 5

Important Research Studies

1) Sickle cell disease

2) Schizophrenia

3) Rheumatoid Arthritis

4) Gastric Cancer

5) Eczema, Psoriasis & Alopecia Areata

6) Sexual Orientation

CHAP. NO. 5

Important Research Studies

Medical scientists have discovered that the hand can be used as an indicator for medical problems. Dermatologists have found that some nail abnormalities communicate reliable information related to health problems. The geneticists have observed that dermatoglyphic aberrations are indicative for certain genetic syndromes (Down's syndrome - mongolism - is the most well-known example). However, other aspects of the hands can signal medical problems as well.

Some research studies have been undertaken in last decade in different countries for medical assessment of some diseases on the basis of different features of human hand. The detail of some studies has been given below, which is equally interested for experts and general readers.

1) Sickle Cell Disease

A research study was undertaken in December 2003, by Dermatology Division, Department of Medicine, University College Hospital, Ibadan, Nigeria for medical assessment of Sickle cell disease on the basis of palmistry. A nexus between sickle cell trait and the extra transverse digital crease on the fingers was studied.

BACKGROUND: Alteration in the location and number of palmar creases has been found in association with certain disorders. The extra transverse digital crease (ETDC) has been reported in sickle cell disease. This study was carried out to determine the importance of ETDC as a diagnostic tool for sickle cell disease.

METHODS: Medical students and student nurses with available hemoglobin electrophoresis records were studied. Their palms were examined for the presence of ETDC.

RESULTS: An ETDC was present in 80 of 178 (44.9%) cases with genotype AA, 26 of 68 (38.2%) cases with sickle cell trait (AS, 65; AC, 3), and 10 of 22 (45.4%) cases with sickle cell disease (SS).

2) Schizophrenia

A research study was undertaken in January 2004, by Department of Psychology, University ELTE, Budapest, Hungary, for medical assessment of schizophrenia on the basis of palmistry. The differentiation of the human brain is triggered by sexual steroid hormones in the fetus. The development of both the urogenital system and the appendicular skeleton are under common control by the HOX genes.

Generally men have longer ring fingers than index fingers, whereas in women these fingers are close to equal.

The inborn digit pattern may reflect fetal estrogen/androgen influences on hemispheric brain specialization. Reduced hemispheric asymmetry has been found in schizophrenia. Gender differences in schizophrenia also suggest a possible endocrine component in the complex pathogenesis of the illness. To test this hypothesis the authors have measured the relative digit lengths of patients with schizophrenia and healthy comparison subjects. The distance of the tip of the index and ring finger was measured from the tip of the third digit in 80 male and 80 female, right-handed patients with DSM-IV diagnosis of schizophrenia and in 80 right-handed healthy comparison men and women.

Schizophrenic men and women showed a more "feminine" phenotype of the index and ring fingers in both hands than same-sex controls. This finding implies that low fetal androgen/estrogen ratio may have a predisposing role in the development of schizophrenia and points toward involvement of endocrine factors in the disturbed   hemispheric   lateralization   attributed   to   the   illness.

3) Rheumatoid Arthritis

A research study was undertaken in October 2003, by Division of Human Genetics, Department of Anatomy St. John's Medical College, Bangalore for medical assessment of rheumatoid arthritis on the basis of palmistry.

Patients with rheumatoid arthritis have been referred to Division of Human Genetics for counseling. Qualitative dermatoglyphics comprising of finger print pattern, interdigital pattern, hypothenar pattern and palmar crease were studied on 26 female and 11 male rheumatoid arthritis patients.

Comparison between patient male and control male; and patient female and control female has been done. 'Chi' square test was performed. In male patients, with hands together, arches were increased, loops/ whorls were decreased. Partial Simian crease was significantly increased.

In the right hand, patterns were increased in the 3rd interdigital area. On the other hand, in female patients there was a significant increase in whorls and decrease in loops on the first finger on both the hands, increase in arches on the 3rd finger; both arches and whorls on the 4th finger of left hand. The study has emphasized that dermatoglyphics could be applied as a diagnostic tool to patients with rheumatoid arthritis.

4) Gastric Cancer

A research study was recently undertaken, by Anesthesiology Department, General Hospital Dr. Ivo Pedisic, Sisak, Croatia for medical assessment of Gastric cancer on the basis of palmistry.

Gastric cancer is very common malignant disease, etiology of that is still unknown. Some studies consider that it is caused by a joint activity of both genetic and environmental factors. Digito-palmar dermatoglyphs were already used to determine hereditary base of some malignant diseases (breast, lung and colorectal cancer) and it was the reason for investigations of the correlation of their quantity features at patients with gastric cancer (36 males and 32 females) and the control groups of phenotypically healthy persons (50 males and 50 females).

By performing statistical data processing of the multivariate and univariate analysis, as well as of discriminant ones, it was possible to prove the existence of heterogeneity between the investigated groups. Higher incidence of gastric cancer and the blood group A could be confirmed, as well.

From the obtained findings it can be concluded, that the results of quantitative analysis of digitopalmar dermatoglyphs affirm the existence of genetic predisposition for development of gastric cancer.

5) Eczema, Psoriasis & Alopecia Areata

A research study was undertaken in August 2003, by Division of Genetics, Medical School, Hamadan, Iran, Department of Genetics and Anthropology, Faculty of Health, Tehran, Iran for medical assessment of eczema, psoriasis and alopecia areata on the basis of palmistry.

BACKGROUND: The study of patterns of fingerprints is important in anthropology and medical genetics, chiefly because of their diagnostic usefulness. In the present work, we studied the frequencies of various types of skin ridges of the first phalanx in patients with eczema, psoriasis and alopecia areata.

METHODS: In a double-blind case-control study, we determined the frequencies of fingerprints in 551 patients (240 cases with eczema, 164 cases with psoriasis and 147 cases with alopecia areata) as well as in general population of Hamadan City (control group: 188 males and 529 females). We compared the frequencies between various fingers, hands and sexes in all three case groups as well as between case groups and control group.

RESULTS: The frequencies of various types of fingerprints are presented in some tables. The results showed that frequencies are not statistically different according to types of fingers, hands (left or right) and sexes as well. But they are significantly different in various case groups and between case groups and control group.

CONCLUSIONS: The frequencies of various patterns of skin ridges differ in eczema, psoriasis and alopecia areata from normal population.

6) Sexual Orientation

Another research study was undertaken in February 2003, Department of Psychiatry, School of Medicine, New York University, New York, New York 10016, USA for medical assessment of sexual orientation on the basis of palmistry.

The second to fourth finger digit ratio (2D:4D ratio) is a sex-dimorphic characteristic in humans that may reflect relative levels of first trimester prenatal sex hormones. Low interdigital ratio has been associated with high levels of androgens. It has been reported in unrelated women that low 2D:4D ratio is associated with lesbian sexual orientation, but because of the nature of those samples, it was not possible to conclude whether lower ratio (and hypothetically, higher androgen levels) in lesbians are due to differences in genetics as opposed to differences in environment.

To test the hypothesis that low 2D:4D in lesbians is due to differences in environment, interdigital ratio data were analyzed in a sample of female monozygotic (MZ) twins discordant for sexual orientation (1 twin was lesbian, the other was heterosexual; n = 7 pairs). A control group of female MZ twins concordant for sexual orientation (both twins were lesbian) was used as a comparison (n = 5 pairs).

In the twins discordant for sexual orientation, the lesbian twins had significantly lower 2D:4D ratios on both the right and left hands than their heterosexual cotwins. There were no significant differences for either hand in the twins concordant for sexual orientation. Because MZ twins share virtually the same genes, differences in 2D:4D ratio suggest that low 2D:4D ratio is a result of differences in prenatal environment.

PART- II

MEDICAL CHIROGNOMY

CHAP: NO. 6

Seven Types of Hand

1. Elementary Hand

2. Conic Hand

3. Square Hand

4. Spatulate Hand

5. Psychic Hand

6. Philosophic Hand

7. Mixed Hand

CHAP NO. 6

Seven Types of Hands

According to the chirognomy, there are seven types of hands:

1. Elementary Hand   2.   Conic Hand.

3. Square Hand.   4.   Spatulate Hand.

5. Psychic Hand.   6.   Philosophic Hand

7. Mixed Hand.

1. Elementary Hand

In appearance, Elementary hand is coarse and clumsy, with large thick heavy palm, short nails, short fingers and short and thick thumb.

An elementary hand indicates lowest type of mentality, lack of intellectual interests, want of imagination and brutal desires. The people with elementary hand are passionate and have a little control over their passions. They are violent in temper. They hate doing mental work or the work requiring mental abilities as they posses a little mental ability and capacity. Such people are more appropriate for the jobs or work requiring physical exercise or labor like boxing, wrestling, factory or industry work and so on.

Generally, the people with elementary hand have a limited scope of life for being deprived of imaginative power. They have animal nature and often they commit serious crimes. If the thumb of a person with elementary hand is extremely short, and simian line (lines of life, head and heart connected together) is found, he may involve in serious crimes like murder torture, kidnapping and terrorism and may rush blindly into danger. If short, swollen and very red mount of Venus is also found, the subject may involve in sexual crimes like rape.

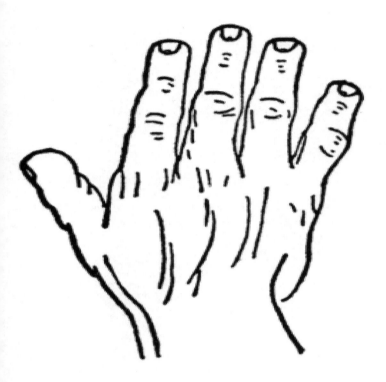

Fig. 6.1 **Elementary Hand**

Criteria for normal Elementary Hand

The elementary hand may be considered as normal from diagnostic point of view if it fulfills the following criteria of normality:

I) A good and straight line of head (better if sloping toward mount of moon in the end) should be present in elementary hand;

II) The thumb of elementary hand should be strong and well developed not weak, short and clubbed;

III) The fourth finger (little finger) should not be ill-formed; and

IV) There should be a good mount of Venus, not exaggerated with unfavorable signs.

A medical palmist should look for unfavorable features or abnormal signs in an elementary hand in order to assess the subject's mental tendencies, which may lead him to some neurotic disorders or psychological complications.

2. Conic Hand

In appearance, conic hand is with palm slightly tapering, the fingers slightly tapering at the tip and full at the base.

A conic hand denotes an artistic temperament, impulsive nature, love of luxury, beauty and indolence, lack of patience and susceptibility to love-affairs. The people with conic hand are generally sensitive, indolent, moody, impulsive, inconstant, sympathetic, nature-loving, emotional, impressionable and quick-tempered. They learn quickly almost everything but they love superficial and subjective study. They may quick in thought but they are devoid of patience and tire easily, that is why, they rarely carry out their intentions.

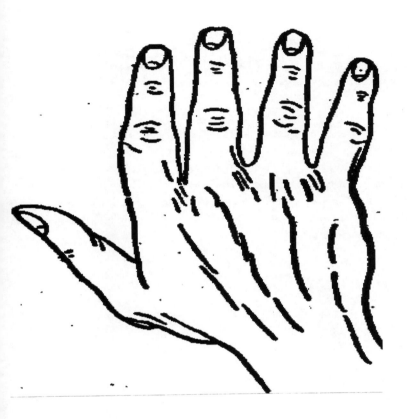

Fig. 6.2 **Conic Hand**

3. Square Hand

In appearance, square hand is square at the wrist, square at the base of fingers and the fingers are themselves square.

Square hand denotes practical nature, force of character, firm-determination, great application in work, love of duties, and firm belief in practicalism. The people with the square hand are practical, punctual and well-principled. They make quick progress in practical life, because they are more hardworking and serious. They love practical study. The people with square hand are sincere in friendship and do their duties with a keen sense of responsibility. They are seen almost in every sphere of life. Their success depend upon their hard-work and pragmatism.

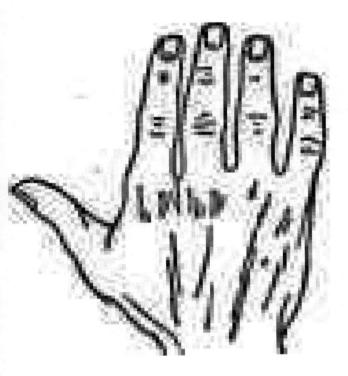

Fig. 6.3   **<u>Square Hand</u>**

4.   Spatulate Hand

The palm of the spatulate hand is either unusually broad at the base of fingers or at the wrist. Each finger of this hand also resembles with spatula.

Spatulate hand denotes energy of purpose, love of action, innovative and inventive mind and a marked individuality of its own.

The people with the spatulate hand have a restless nature. They are enthusiastic and have intense love of independence. Spatulate hand belongs to the great discoverers, explorers, engineers and great inventors.

Such people are full with vital force. They make policies and schemes with their imaginative and inventive mind. They use their talents for making useful things of life. They are true realist and creative and they accept the challenges of life.

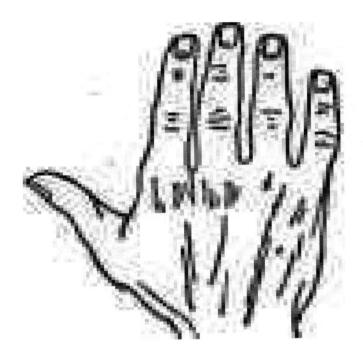

Fig. 6.4   **Spatulate Hand**

5. Philosophic Hand

In appearance, philosophic hand is long angular with long fingers, developed joints and long nails.

The people with the philosophic hand have a philosophical nature. They are silent, secretive, ambitious, thoughtful, distinctive, careful over minute matters and argumentative characters. Such people love mystery in all things. They have a great tendency towards reading, writing and literature. They love isolation from the world and often they happen to be religious minded. They feel pride of being isolated and different from others.

The people with the philosophic hand have a great power of analysis. They are deep thinkers and they do not accept anything without arguments and logic.

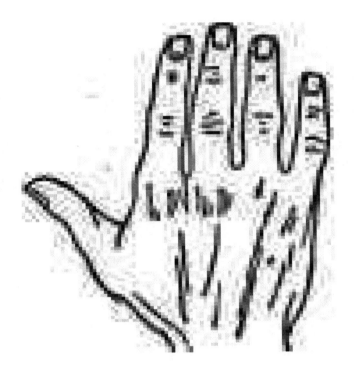

Fig. 6.5   **Philosophic Hand**

6. Psychic Hand

In appearance, psychic hand is long with slender tapering fingers and long almond shaped nails.

People with the psychic hand have an idealistic nature but they have no idea of how to be practical. They are easily influenced by others and they trust every one who is kind to them. They live in the world of dreams and they do not aware of the practical aspects of life. They are highly sensitive and often they fall victim of inferiority complex. They have great attraction for magic and mystery. If the first phalange of the thumb of this hand is shorter than the first, then such people may live in fool's paradise.

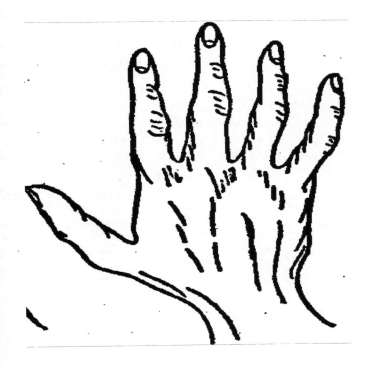

Fig. 6.6   **Psychic Hand**

7. **Mixed Hand**

This hand is the mixture of seven types. It can not be classed as conic, square, spatulate, psychic or philosophic; the fingers also belong to different types- often one conic, one square, one psychic etc.

The mixed hand denotes versatility and changeability of ideas, diplomacy and tact, adaptability to men and circumstances and restless nature. The people with the mixed hand are clever but erratic in application of their talents. Such people can talk on every subject or topic of the life but they cannot impress other people with the depth of their ideas and thought. They have no difficulty in getting on with the different dispositions with which they come in contact. Their most striking peculiarity is their adaptability to circumstances, as they are always changing with circumstances. Truly speaking, they may be called as "jack of all trades but master of none".

If the head-line in a mixed hand is straight, then it is possible that, such a person will choose the best one of all his talents and succeed.

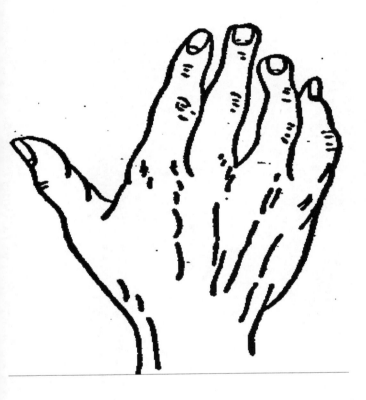

Fig. 6.7   **Mixed Hand**

CHAP: NO.7

Nails

1- Normal Criteria for Nails

2- Diagnosis of Diseases through Analysis of Nails

a) Heart Disease and Blood Circulation

b) Nervous Diseases

c) Chest & Lung Diseases

d) Other Diseases

CHAP: NO.7

Nails

Nails of the fingers are the most important area of medical palmistry. They provide guidance about health problems. The nails are considered as the 'diagnostic screens' where different signs and different colors indicate different physical and psychic disorders. While collecting palmistic data for the diagnosis of some disease, these diagnostic screens with different signs are carefully analyzed. Nails wonderfully indicate not only about a person's disease, but they also predict the diseases, he may prone. Besides diseases, the nails also reveal the disposition and temperament. Generally, the people with short nails are more critical than those of with long nails. Habit of biting nails indicates a nervous temperament.

Medical Science has demonstrated that, the nail of Jupiter's Finger (First Finger) belongs to the hepatic faculties. So a number of quite important indications of liver disorders like jaundice etc. can be observed through the first finger's nail. Similarly, nail of Saturn's finger (second finger) belongs to skeleton, nail of Sun's finger (third) to cardiorenal faculties and nail of mercury's finger (fourth) belongs to the nervous system. Therefore, keeping this medical information about nails, readers can predict a person's diseases, especially those of liver, kidneys, heart, nerves and spinal chord.

Criteria for Normal Nails

Criterion for normal nails is described as follows:

I)   The nails should be free from unfavorable signs such as spots, dots, and ridges.

II)   Moons on the nails must be of normal size, neither very large nor very small.

III)   The nails must not appear to be sunken into the flesh at the base or inclined to curve out at edges.

IV)   The nails must not be of white, blue, or of deep red color.

2- Diagnosis of Diseases through Analysis of Nails

Different formations, colors, and types of nails and their careful analysis may lead a medical pamist to the diagnosis of many diseases. It has been demonstrated by the medical science that diagnosis of a large number of diseases like heart disease, nervous disease, lung disease, throat disease and so on, is possible through deep study of nails.

From the early 1980's, various works have been published which describe the clinical relevance of the nails. A classical example in this field is the work presented by Beaven & Brooks: Color Atlas of the Nail in Clinical Diagnosis (first print: 1984). In the past years various new books have been presented within this discipline.

However, only a few years ago medical students were hardly informed about the clinical value of the nails. In order to fill this space several dermatologists have united their knowledge. In 1997, they created 'Nail-TutorTM': a visual personal computer program including 150 photos, which describe the anatomy and pathology of the nails - afterwards the user can test the understanding of the material in the program. (www.handresearch.com)

Now I would like to illustrate how we can diagnose diseases through nails. While predicting diseases through examination of nails the normal criteria for nails must be kept in mind.

A) Heart Disease & Blood Circulation

The following indications and symptoms of weak heart and poor circulation of blood can be observed on the nails:

I) Blueness at the base of any nail indicates a weak heart and poor circulation of blood.

II) When blueness is observed at the base of small tapering nails with the end quite square, and tapering towards the base, it means pronounced heart trouble.

III) At the base of the nail there is a curved white portion, which is called as moon.

a) Small moons indicate weak action of heart and poor circulation of blood.

b) Large moons indicate rapid circulation of blood and a strong action of heart.

c) Very large of the moons on the nails denotes much pressure on the heart.

d) The nails without moons show an advanced stage of the disease.

IV) Conical nails indicate poor physical health and poor blood circulatory system.

V) If long nails are bluish in color and are wider at the top, the poor blood circulation will be the result.

VI) If blueness is found on the nails at the age of 12 to 14 years, it would be temporary obstruction of blood circulation and would not be taken as serious one. But if blueness is found at the age of 18 to 42 years it indicates serious trouble. When it is again found at the age of 43 to 47 it denotes a difficulty of probably short duration.

VII) Short and pale nails indicate anemia, and physical weakness.

B) Nervous Diseases

Following indications or symptoms can be observed on the nails of a nervous patient:

I) The brittle and fluted nails indicate nervous disease. Therefore, the nails from top to the base must be smooth and not composed of ridges or flutings as the ridges or flutings of nails from top to the base is an indication of nervous disorder.

II) When the nails are short and are very flat and sunk into flesh at the base they indicate nervous disorders.

III) White spots or dots on the nails denote nervous disease and also denote advanced stage of nervous break-down.

IV) Cross-ridges on the nails are another indication of nervousness.

V) Appearance of white dots on the nails is the first warning of delicate nerves, beginning of loss of vitality and a complete medical check-up under such indications is inevitable.

VI) Short nails, which are very flat and inclined to curve out at the edges, indicate symptoms of paralysis.

VII) V - Shaped nails indicate some nervous disease.

C) Chest & Lung Diseases

I) Curved nails indicate delicacy of bronchial tubes and weakness of lungs.

II) Clubbed nails denote the indications of tuberculosis and lung disease.

II) Very long-nailed persons may prone to chest and lung disease.

D) Other Diseases

I) Black or bluish spots on the nails denote blood poisoning.

II) Very short and round shaped nails indicate an anxious temperament.

III) Sometimes, V-shaped nails indicate throat trouble.

IV) Delicate and narrow nails is an indication of a delicate constitution

V) Narrow nails indicate lack of muscular strength.

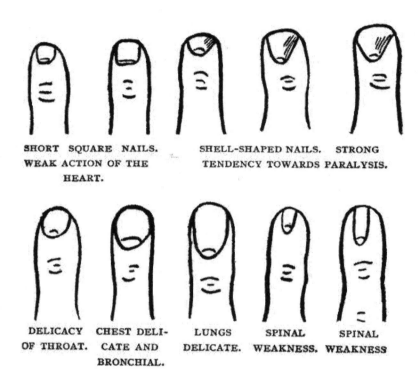

SHORT SQUARE NAILS.   SHELL-SHAPED NAILS.   STRONG
WEAK ACTION OF THE   TENDENCY TOWARDS PARALYSIS.
HEART.

DELICACY   CHEST DELI-   LUNGS   SPINAL   SPINAL
OF THROAT.   CATE AND   DELICATE.   WEAKNESS.   WEAKNESS
           BRONCHIAL.

Fig. 7.1 **Different Shapes of Nails**

CHAP: NO.8

Palm & Hair

1- Diagnosis of Diseases through Analysis of Palm

a) Thyroid Secretion & Palm

b) Other Diseases

2- Hair Growing on Hands

CHAP: NO. 8

Palm & Hair

There are more nerves in the palm than any other portion of the hand. Medical Science has also demonstrated that the palm of the hand is under the control and actions of the nerves or nerve fluid. Naturally, the palm of the hand is covered by a fine skin, which may vary in color in various hands.

1- Diagnosis of Diseases Through Analysis of Palm

Different types of diseases can be diagnosed through a careful examination of palm, its color and the different signs on the skin of the palm. Therefore, the analysis of palm, in the medical palmistry, is of great importance.

a) Thyroid Secretion & Palm

Thyroid glands are important endocrine glands, which are located in the thorax in the form of a pair. Thyroids secrete two important hormones i.e. (I) Thyroxin   (II) Calcitonin.

I) Thyroxin increases the rate of chemical reactions in almost all the cells of the body, which results in the increase of rate of the body metabolism.

II) Calcitonin increases the use of calcium in the bones and thus decreases calcium concentration from tissue fluid.

Therefore, the decrease or increase in the rate of thyroid secretion may result in serious physical disorders. These disorders which are caused by over or less activity of thyroid glands can be observed in the hands, as under:

1. A soft, warm and moist skin of the palm indicates over-activity of thyroid glands.

2. If the skin is dry and scaly, it indicates less-activity of thyroid glands.

b) Other Diseases

A number of diseases can be diagnosed through a careful analysis of skin of the palm as follows:

I) When the palm of the hand is yellowish in color, it indicates intestinal disorders like dyspepsia, and defect in parastalysis.

II) If the palm of the hand is pale, it shows sickness and bloodlessness.

III) If the palm is blue, it indicates biloiusness. The blue color of palm also indicates poor circulation of blood.

IV) When the color of the palm is white, it indicates lack of blood supply and lack of red blood cells (RBCs) in the blood. However, in the hand of a woman, whiteness is natural which does not indicate physical disorders.

V) Pink color of the palm indicates good health with normal function of heart and a blood rich in red corpuscles, energy and vitality.

2- Hair Growing on Hands

In the medical palmistry, the hairs growing on the hand also provide us with useful mental and physical conditions of a person.

Cheiro presents a suggested theory about hair, which is stated as below:

"Each hair is in itself fine tube: These tubes are in connection with the skin and skin nerves. Through these hair or tubes escape the nervic electricity of the body, and by the color they take passage of that electricity. The flow of this electricity through the hair makes the hair black, brown, blond, gray or white".

Hairs of different colors reveal different dispositions, temperament and nature which help the medical palmist in diagnosis of psychological disorders of a subject.

1) Blond Hair

The people with the blond or Brown hair are very gentle by nature as the less quantity of electricity escape through tubes (hairs).

2) Dark Hair

People with very dark hair have more passion in temper, and are more irritable and more energetic in affection, than those of with the blond hair.

3) Red Hair

The people with the red hair have greater quantity of electricity and due to having greater supply and force of electricity they are more excitable.

4) White Hair

The white hairs on the hand are very rarely seen. White hair denotes nervous diseases, especially 'Shock.' This is because of the fact that, the hair is connected with the nerves of the skin and the force of the nervous electric fluid is rushing through these hairs. When this nervous electric fluid system gets old on account of aging, this fluid is not generated in large quantities and as a result, hair begins to grow white.

CHAP: NO.9

Thumb

CHAP: NO.9

Thumb

Thumb reveals three important powers of a person i-e will, logic and love. The first phalange (nail phalange) of thumb indicates will power, second phalange denotes logic and third (boundary of mount of Venus) the love. While strength of will and force of character is indicated by a long thumb, and a weak will power is denoted by a short thumb.

1- Phalanges of Thumb

I. First Phalange

Besides will power, the first phalange of thumb also denotes a subject's power of decision, power of competition and his perseverance. The people with extremely long first phalange of thumb depend neither upon logic nor reason but they simply depend upon will. A very small first phalange indicates a weak force of character, lack of self-confidence and weakness of will.

II. Second Phalange

The second phalange of thumb denotes logic and arguing capability. If the second phalange is longer than the first, the subject will have the capacity to do long discussions but will lack strength of will and force of decision.

III. Third Phalange

The third phalange (mount of Venus) of thumb denotes not only love but also the sensuality, passion and sex-urge. If it is short, developed and red in color, it indicates less control over passions, sensual desires and lasciviousness.

2- Freud Theory & Thumb

SIGMUND Freud has laid great stress on sex and unconscious force in his theory about personality. Freud has divided the human mind into three areas or forces:

I. Id   II. Ego   III. Super Ego.

I. ID

It is unconscious area of mind, which is replete with carnal desires, animal passions, sex-urge and innate or natural proclivities toward saturation of sensual pleasures. In fact, Id is a blind force that wants saturation of its innate appetites at any cost.

II. EGO

This is the controlling and also erasing faculty of mind. It controls the passions, carnality, lasciviousness and sensual appetites of id and makes it in consonance with external environment and requirement or circumstances.

Ego logically measures the Id's blind desires and put them under censorship. It lays the foundation of a person's social behavior and moral character.

III. SUPER EGO.

This is regarded as 'Social conscience.' Superego is the highest rung of the ladder of consciousness, intellect and wisdom. It makes the person realize his sins or mistakes and appreciates him for his good deeds.

Thumb may be interpreted as human mind (in accordance with FRUED theory) with three areas or forces. The three phalanges of thumb may be interpreted as three areas of human mind.

1.   Third phalange (mount of Venus) may be interpreted as Id.

2.   Second phalange as Ego; and

3.   First phalange as superego.

I)   Third Phalange (ID)

Third phalange of thumb which is a boundary of mount of Venus denotes 'love'. It is an established fact that love is considered a blind passion that is devoid of any reason or rationale, as it concerns with passion, emotion and heart's desire.

Third phalange like 'ID' denotes sensuality, sex-urge, passions, carnal desires and innate proclivities of a person toward gratification of sensual pleasures. The texture, shape and size of the third phalange reveal the magnitude and intensity of passionate force emanating from ID. A careful analysis of third phalange of thumb may lead to prediction of a subject's baser instincts, sensual appetites, sex-urge and the disorders resulting from the gravity of such passions and instincts.

II. Second Phalange (EGO)

Second phalange of thumb denotes logic. According to Freud, Ego controls the Id's sensual appetites and provides logic for their satisfaction. Ego is a nexus between Id's appetites and super-Ego's requirements with reference to the external conditions. Second phalange of thumb like ego denotes the reasoning faculty of mind.

III. First Phalange (SUPER EGO)

First phalange of thumb denotes will power and force of decision. Super ego which is the highest place of consciousness, intellect and wisdom, takes the final decision about a subject's intention, plan or scheme. First phalange like super ego denotes a subject's power of decision in view of the external conditions and circumstances.

3- Types of Thumb

There are two types of thumb:

I) Supple-Jointed thumb

II) Firm-Jointed thumb.

I) Supple-jointed Thumb

A supple-jointed thumb denotes lack of will power, freedom of thought, adaptability of temperament, extravagance in matters of money, pleasant but flexible nature and lack of energy of purpose.

2) Firm-jointed Thumb

Firm-Jointed thumb denotes stability in ideas, stubborn determination,

strength of will, force of character, and energy of purpose.

2) Clubbed Thumb

It is so called because of its club-like shape. It is thick from the upper side, thinner from the center and again thick from the end. The tip of the thumb is fleshy and the thumbnail is short and broad. The clubbed thumb denotes a strong will, brutal obstinacy and a powerful but violent temper, which may lead the subject to kill someone.

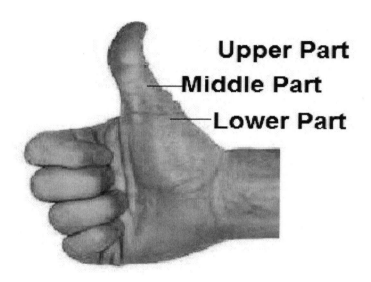

Fig. 9.1   **Phalenges of Thumb**

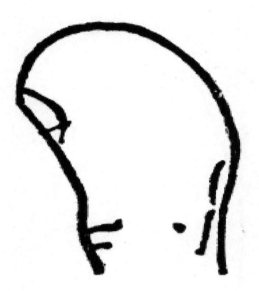

Fig. 9.2   **Clubbed Thumb**

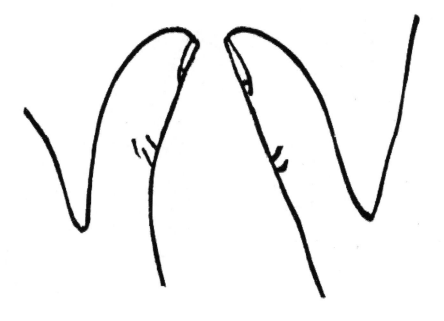

Fig. 9.3   **<u>Supple & firm-jointed Thumbs</u>**

CHAP: NO. 10

Fingers

CHAP: NO. 10

Fingers

From diagnostic point of view, the fingers of hand provide a profile of a subject's materialistic, spiritualistic, imaginative, idealistic and mental faculties. Therefore, fingers are of immense importance in the field of medical palmistry.

1. The first finger or index finger is called as finger of Jupiter;

2. Second finger is called as finger of Saturn;

3. Third finger is called as finger of sun; and

4. Fourth finger is called as finger of mercury.

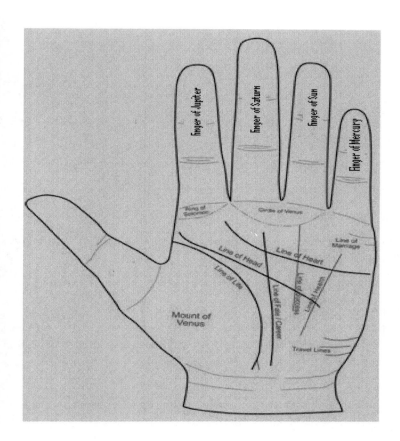

Fig. 10.1 **Fingers of hand**

1- **Finger of Jupiter**

The finger of Jupiter denotes power to rule and to command over people. It should not be excessively long or short but it should be long with normal features.

Criteria for Normal Jupiter-Finger

A finger of Jupiter is considered as normal if it fulfills the following criteria:-

I) In length, the finger of Jupiter should extend to the mid-line of the first phalange of the second finger. This is the normal length of finger of Jupiter.

II) The finger of Jupiter should not be appreciably shorter than the finger of sun.

III) The finger of Jupiter should not be longer than the "normal length."

IV)   The finger should not be crooked.

Now by applying the rule, "Anything beyond normal is abnormal", a medical palmist can reach the following conclusions:

I) If the finger of Jupiter is exceptionally long, it denotes a haughty, aggressive, tyrannical, arrogant and over-confident subject.

II) If the finger of Jupiter is short (shorter than normal) it denotes inferiority complex, lack of self-confidence, dislike of responsibility, and inability to face the challenges of life. Such a subject may fall victim of frustration and despondency and may prone to hypertension and other nervous disorders.

III) A crooked finger of Jupiter denotes lack of principle in rule and ambition.

2. **Finger of Saturn**

The finger of Saturn denotes thoughtfulness, love of solitude and carefulness in thought and action and also tendencies towards pessimism, melancholy and retardation.

Finger of Saturn is also called as middle finger because it establishes a 'balance' between conscious and unconscious, active and passive and physical and mental aspects of one's life. An exceptionally long or excessively short finger of Saturn will be considered to be an abnormal finger as it will disturb this balance leading a person to some sort of illness.

Criteria for Normal Saturn-Finger

A finger of Saturn is considered to be normal if it fulfills the following criteria:

I) A finger of Saturn should not be exceptionally long.

II) It should not be short (almost equal to the third finger) and pointed.

III) It should not be ill-formed or crooked.

The Medical palmist can conclude:-

I) A very long finger of Saturn will show morbid desires, melancholy and a pessimistic behavior. A person with very long finger of Saturn may prone to retardation and pessimism which may lead him to isolation from the world or to suicide ultimately (if other unfavorable signs are also present in hand).

II) If the finger of Saturn is very short and pointed it denotes frivolity.

III) A crooked finger of Saturn denotes extreme sensitiveness and a morbid nature. Such a person may have tendencies toward suicide especially if the line of head is sloping toward mount of moon and reaching near the wrist.

VI) A medical palmist should also note the bending nail phalange toward finger of sun which points to some intestinal disorders. However before making an assessment some other signs of intestinal disorders from the hand must be confirmed.

3. Finger of Sun

The finger of sun denotes a person's artistic talent, his ambitions for honor, glory and fame and his love of art. This finger is considered of great importance in the field of medical palmistry, as it is believed that heart is connected with it by an artery. A normal finger of sun reveals a normal function of heart (if other signs are also favorable in the hand) and an abnormal finger may be taken as a sign of cardiovascular complications.

Criteria for Normal Sun-Finger

I) The finger of sun should be of normal length i.e. not almost equal to the finger of Saturn and not very shorter than the finger of Jupiter.

II) It should not be crooked.

III) It should not appear to be bending inward over the palm.

IV)   The finger of sun should not lean toward finger of Saturn.

A careful analysis of finger of sun may lead the medical palmist to the following conclusions:-

I)   A crooked finger of sun is a sign of heart disease.

II) If it bends inward over the palm it denotes emotional disturbance and a weak function of heart.

III)   An excessively long finger of sun reveals a state of utopia and a craving for notoriety.

IV)   If it is leaning towards finger of Saturn, it denotes morbid sensitiveness.

V)   If it is very short, it reveals dislike to publicity.

4. Finger of Mercury

The finger of mercury reveals a subject's power of expression, diplomacy, mental power, behavioral deviation, and problems in his personal relationship with opposite sex or with others and also his propensities toward uterine disorders.

Criteria for Normal Mercury-Finger

I) A mercury finger should be of normal length i.e. extending almost to the mid-line of the first phalange of finger of sun.

II)   It should not appear as 'distorted' one.

III)   The nail-phalange of the finger should not bend inward over the palm.

VI)   The phalanges should be free from unfavorable signs.

V)   The finger of mercury should not seem to be separated from other fingers.

An analysis of finger of mercury may lead the medical palmist to the following conclusions:-

1. An excessively long finger of mercury denotes diplomacy of extreme degree and a great power to influence and to convince people through deceptive talk.

2. A very short finger of mercury denotes lack of sharpness of mind in grasping some ideas and lack of expression either in words or writing. A very short finger also arises suspicion

about a person's character, particularly when other unfavorable signs in the hand will also be found.

3. A distorted finger of mercury signifies trickery and a devilish mentality. Such a finger sometimes indicates a genetic disorder of thyroid secretion (often less-activity of thyroid glands).

4. When the finger of mercury seems to be isolated from other fingers, it denotes some sort of inner conflict going on in the personal relationship of a person with others especially with opposite sex. Such a finger points to the dissatisfaction of the subject with his married life.

5. The finger of mercury is believed to be connected with urino-genital system. If the third phalange of this finger is thick and a deep vertical line is cutting the second phalange; it is a sign of urino-genital disorder.

6. If the nail phalange of the finger of mercury appears to be bending inward over palm, it reveals renal disorders.

7. Deviate behaviors involving inclinations toward criminal pursuits and sexual abuse are indicated by an abnormal finger of mercury when it is short and twisted. However, while making an assessment a careful analysis of mount of Venus, head-line, heart-line and thumb should be made.

5. Types of Fingers

Different types of fingers are analyzed as follows:

I.   **Short Fingers**

Short fingers denote dislike of detail, quickness in thought and action and lack of analyzing power. The people with short fingers are impulsive, quick, and conclusive. They love conciseness and preciseness in everything.

II.   **Long Fingers**

Long fingers denote love of detail, power of analysis, and restlessness about little things. The people with long fingers like detail in everything. They may be troubled over minute things. They remain engaged in deliberating and concentrating on minor things.

III.   **Knotty Fingers**

Knotty fingers denote analytical mind, thoughtfulness and a philosophical nature.

IV.   **Thick Fingers**

Thick fingers denote materialism, desire for luxury and comforts of life.

V.   **Thin Fingers**

Thin fingers reveal spiritual qualities and a control over materialistic desires

VI.   **Soft Fingers**

Soft fingers denote rashness in everything and a less critical nature.

CHAP: NO. 11

Mounts of the Hand

1. Mount of Jupiter

2. Mount of Saturn

3. Mount of Sun

4. Mount of Mercury

5. Mount of Venus

6. Mount of Moon

7. First Mount of Mars (POSITIVE)

8. Second Mount of Mars (NEGATIVE)

9 Mount of Neptune

CHAP: NO. 11

Mounts of the Hand

The study of mounts of the hand is important area of medical palmistry. The mounts are the slight elevations on the palm. Each mount is constituted by pulpy tissue. It is the nerve-terminal in the bundle of muscles wreathing the palm. The mounts are believed to have some pathological correlates, as their abnormal or deficient development reveals a person's hereditary ailments and also provides a profile of his physical, psychological, emotional, spiritual and mental make-up. Depth of the palm is determined by the excessive or depressive development of the mounts. The mounts of the hand are considered to be the reservoirs of nervous fluid. They also help the hand tighten its grip, like cushions, around a thing.

Normal Criteria for Mounts

1. A mount should not appear to be 'depressed.'

2. A mount should not be excessively developed or grown.

Mounts of the Hand

1. Mount of Jupiter

It is situated at the base of first finger.

2. Mount of Saturn

It is found at the root of second finger.

3. Mount of Sun

It is found at the root of third finger.

4. Mount of Mercury

It is located at the base of fourth finger.

5. Mount of Venus

It is found at the base of thumb.

6. Mount of Moon

It is found at just above the bracelets, near the percussion.

7.   First Mount of Mars (POSITIVE)

It is found near the line of life and close to the head-line.

8.   Second Mount of Mars (NEGATIVE)

It is found between line of head and line of heart, close to the percussion and under the mount of mercury.

9. Mount of Neptune

This mount is situated in between the mount of Venus and mount of moon.

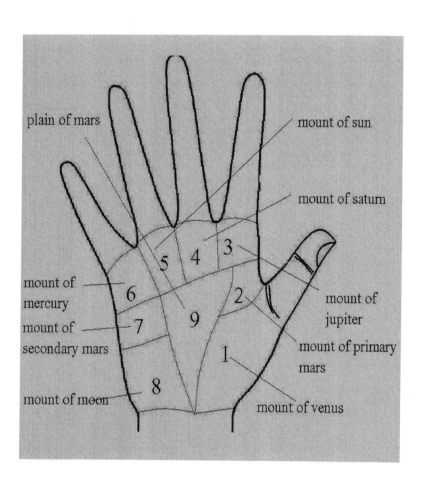

Fig. 11.1   **Mounts of Hand**

1) Mount of Jupiter

A well-developed and good mount of Jupiter denotes pride, dignity, and desire for power, generosity, leadership, principle, honor and a sympathetic attitude toward other people.

When this mount is found to be in "depressed" form, it reveals lack of commanding capabilities and self-respect. Such a person may have a selfish nature and sensual desires.

When this mount appears to be excessively developed, it denotes egotism, intense love of power, haughtiness, and a strong desire to command.

When the mount of Jupiter is ruling over all other mounts in the hand, the person is named as jupiterian. The jupiterians are fond of eating, drinking and may prone to digestive disorders.

2) Mount of Saturn

The mount of Saturn denotes love of solitude, love of philosophy and occult sciences, sobriety and prudence. When this mount is very low or depressed it reveals tendencies of the person toward despondency and pessimism which resultantly lead him to some disease.

When the mount is excessively developed, it denotes morbid melancholy, depression and extreme sensitiveness.

The mount of Saturn is associated with the skeletal and nervous disorders, which are indicated by a bad mount with bad signs.

A saturnine may prone to insanity and subject to varicose veins.

3) Mount of Sun

Mount of sun denotes love of art, beauty, glory and creative talents. When this mount appears to be depressed, it denotes indifferentism to art. If the mount is excessively developed, it reveals self-deception, love of show-off and great pride. A solar person may prone to optic and cardiac troubles.

4) Mount of Mercury

Mount of mercury reveals a person's power of expression, ability to influence others, intellectual powers and quickness in thought.

When the mount is deficient, it denotes deficiency of literary talents and intellectual power. A Mercurian may have a nervous temperament and may prone to digestive and nervous disorders.

5) Mount of Venus

The mount of Venus represents a person's loving nature, sensuality, vitality, animal passions, sex-urge and his libidinous tendencies. The region of Venus is considered to be the vital portion of hand wreathed by the great palmer arch and several nerves in the hand and thus there is a greater flow of blood through this larger blood vessel and a greater flow of nervic-current through the nerves. Therefore, warmth of heart and feelings, physical vitality, robust health and a passionate nature is indicated by a well-developed and good mount of Venus.

If the mount of Venus is excessively developed, elevated, red and hard (with other unfavorable signs in the hand), it denotes excess of debauchery, sensuality, animal passions, and libidinous tendencies. Such an excess may lead the subject to the diseases linked with sexual and sensual abuses like venereal and psychic disorders.

When the mount of Venus is found as depressed or deficient, it indicates coldness of heart and feelings, deficient sex-urge, poor health and cold nature.

6) Mount of Moon

The mount of moon represents the unconscious part of our mind which stores memory, hidden fright and deep feelings. It denotes imagination, romance, idealism, fancy, superstition, intuition and love of imaginative literature.

When the mount of moon is weak and depressed, it denotes a dry nature, lack of creative and imaginative faculties, and lack of romantic feelings.

If the mount is excessively developed and higher than the mount of Venus, it denotes daydreaming, restlessness, irritability, and love of solitude. The mount of moon reveals a person's propensities toward nervous disorders, psychological "complexes" and also the troubles of kidneys and urinary bladder.

7) First Mount of Mars

First mount of mars denotes fighting courage, resistance against attack, vital force, energy of purpose, perseverance, self-reliance and a desire for martial life. When this mount is excessively developed, it denotes recalcitrance to restraints, aggressive behavior and a violent character. Such a subject is full of vital energy and may prone to diseases like stroke, high blood pressure, palpitation of heart and heart-attack resulting from his aggressive and violent behavior and over-excitement.

When the first mount of mars is deficient it indicates timidity, lack of resistive force, and a weak will-power. A Martian possesses a robust health and great resistance against diseases of all kinds. Such a person possesses considerable immunity against fatal infections.

8) Second Mount of Mars

A well-developed second mount of mars indicates moral courage, mental power, strong will-power, martial talents, steadfastness and a strong resistance to mental stress. When this mount is excessively developed, it denotes a violent temperament, zealous nature and stubbornness in opposition. When the second mount of mars is deficient it denotes lack of moral courage, mental retardation and a weak determination.

9) Mount of Neptune

The mount of Neptune represents a balance between lunarian (moon's) characteristics and characteristics associated with Venus and indicates a pleasant disposition, magnetic personality, and powers of expression and impression.

PART III

MEDICAL CHIROMANCY

CHAP: NO.12

Lines & Signs on Palm

1) Color of Lines

2) Different Formations of Lines

3) Principal Lines of Hand

4) Diagnostic Lines

5) Reference-Lines

6) Different Signs

CHAP: NO.12

Lines & Signs on Palm

As earlier stated, lines of the hand are analyzed to assess the pathological correlates in the branch of palmistry known as medical chiromancy. A medical palmist must be fully aware of the criteria for normal color, formation, location, position and appearance of lines on the palm. Keeping in mind the normality criterion for each (principal) line, he can apply the rule, "anything beyond normal is abnormal", for making an assessment. However, before predicting a disease, the medical palmist should review carefully the cheirognomy of hand i.e examination of nails, fingers, palm, and type of the hand.

90

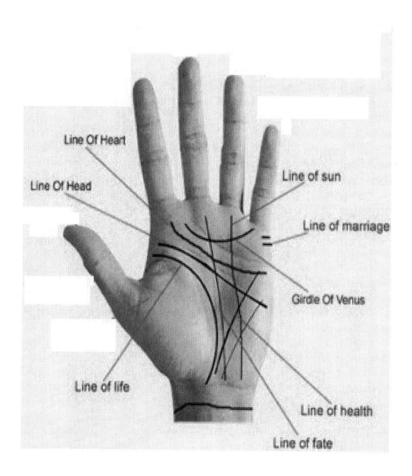

Fig. 12.1 **Major Lines of Hand**

1- Color of Lines

Generally, the lines of following different colors appear on the palm of hand:

I) Red Lines

When the lines appearing to be red in color, the subject will have a robust temperament. Such a person may prone to high blood pressure.

II) Yellow Lines

When lines are yellow in color, the subject will have a bilious temperament. Such a person may prone to hepatic disorders.

III) Pale Lines

Pale lines indicate lack of vitality, poor circulation of blood and deficiency of red blood cells in the blood. The subject is likely to suffer from gastric disorders.

IV) Dark Lines

When the lines are dark in color, the subject will have a somber temperament. Such a person may prone to gastritis.

V) Pink Lines

Pink is considered to be the normal color of lines, as it indicates a robust health with a good circulation of blood, nervous energy and physical strength.

2) Different Formations of Lines

Lines appear on the palm in following different forms:-

I) Broad & Shallow lines

Broad and shallow lines denote desire for sensual pleasures, animal passions, low mental capacity, and psycho-physical weakness.

II)   Intricate lines

When a network of fine lines is found in the hand, it indicates a worrying and highly nervous temperament. Such a person will have a troubled nature and may prone to anxiety, phobia, and other psychosomatic complications.

III)   Wavy lines

Wavy lines denote weakness, inconsistency, and instability of purpose. Such a person will lack the energy to carry out mental pursuits. Wavy lines also indicate insufficient flow of nervic electricity.

IV)   Chained lines

Chained lines indicate obstructions, loss of nervous energy and a poor health.

V)   Thin lines

Thin lines denote lack of physical strength but more nervous energy.

VI)   Thick lines

Thick lines denote lack of nervous energy but more physical strength.

3) Principal Lines of Hand

The principal lines and their location and position in the hand are as follows:-

I)   Line of vitality or Line of Life

A circular line embracing the mount of Venus under the thumb is called as line of vitality or life-line.

II)   Line of Head

It starts under the mount of Jupiter i.e. from the first mount of mars and reaches the second mount of mars. It crosses the center of the hand, horizontally dividing the hand into two parts.

III) Line of Heart

The line of heart commences from under the finger of mercury (below the mount of mercury) and runs toward the mount of Jupiter.

IV)   **Line of Health**

It runs from the mount of mercury (under the fourth finger) down the hand.

V)   **Line of Saturn**

It starts from wrist and reaches the mount of Saturn.   It is also called as fate-line.

VI)   **Line of Sun**

It normally rises from plain of mars and goes toward mount of sun.

VII)   **Line of Mars**

It rises from first mount of mars and runs parallel to and within line of life.   It is also called as inner life-line.

VIII)   **Line of Intuition**

It is a semi-circular line starting from mount of Mercury and ending at mount of moon.

IX)   **Girdle of Venus**

It is a line encircling mounts of Saturn and sun, and found above the line of heart.

X)   **Bracelets**

There are, normally, three bracelets found on the wrist.

4) Diagnostic Lines

A medical palmist's chief interest lies in making an assessment about a person's health, so he should pay greater heed to the analysis of lines which provide a profile of his physical, mental and psychological ailments. The lines which are most important from diagnostic point of view are named as diagnostic lines in the medical palmistry which have direct pathological correlates.

Diagnostic lines include:

I)   Line of vitality

II)   Line of head

III)   Line of heart

III)   Line of health.

5) **Reference-Lines**

The lines which are indirectly related to the disease and refer to the circumstances or problems in confrontation of what the subject may fall prey to some illness, are called as reference lines. Important reference lines include:

1-   Line of Saturn

2.   Line of Sun

3.   Line of Mars

4.   Girdle of Venus

5.   Line of intuition

6.   Via Lasciva

7-   Three bracelets

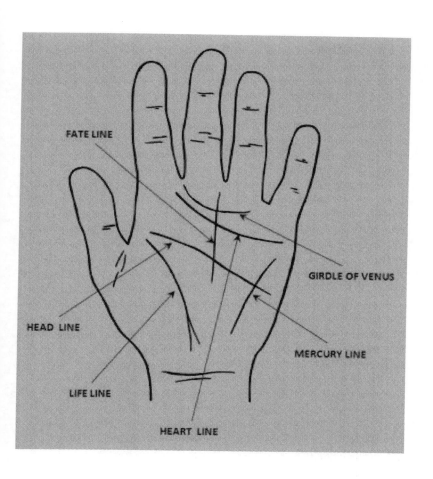

Fig. 12.2 **Reference Lines**

6) Different Signs

Generally following are the different signs which appear on the palm of hand:-

1. Cross   2. Island

3. Square   4. Triangle

5. Star   6. Dots or Spots

7. Circle

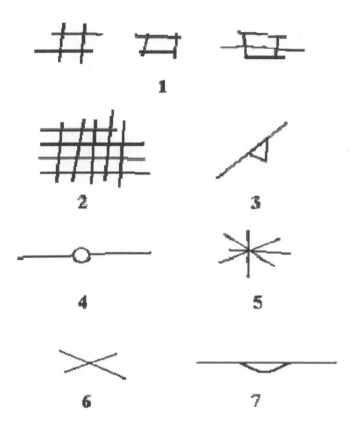

1. Square, 2. Bar, 3. Triangle, 4. Circle, 5. Star, 6. Cross, 7. Island.

Fig. 12.3 **Signs on Palm**

CHAP: NO.13

LINE OF HEALTH

The line of health is the chief diagnostic line whose analysis is of immense importance for the practitioners of medical palmistry. It is generally known line of liver, as it indicates the working condition of liver. The line also indicates the hepatic disorders caused by any defect in the normal function of the liver.

Liver has anatomic proximity with biliary tract and pancreas and also closely interrelated to them in functions. The intermediary metabolism of all foodstuffs occurs here. Liver secretes bile which is a greenish fluid and plays an important role in the digestion of fats. It has an enormous reserve capacity and most of the synthetic, catabolic and detoxifying activities of the body take place here. So liver is one of the most frequently injured organs of the body.

When normal function of liver is disturbed, it disturbs the working condition of many organs of the body, functionally associated with it, causing the body to suffer possibly from digestive, hepatic, pancreatic, nervous or various other disorders. So abnormal working condition of liver can badly affect the health of the whole body.

The line of liver not only denotes the working condition of the liver and disorders of liver, but also represents the health of entire-body indicating various diseases, the body may suffer. Hence, this line has rightly been called as line of health.

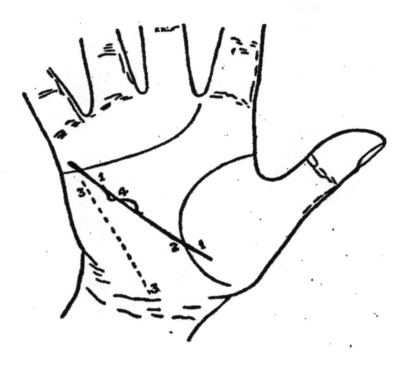

Fig. 13.1 **Line of Health**

Criteria for Normal Health-line

A medical palmist must keep in mind that absence of this line in the hand indicates a good health. However, when it appears on the palm, it must fulfill the criteria for its normality regarding its position, appearance, formation and location.

Normal location & position

The line of health normally arises from mount of mercury and goes down the hand approaching the line of vitality. The line of health should not touch the line of vitality.

Normal Formation & Appearance

Line of health should be free from all defects. It should be straight running down the hand (without touching line of vitality), deep, even and unbroken.

A normal formation of the line will be free of all breaks, cuttings and also of unfavorable signs like islands, dots, crossbars etc.

The line of health should not appear either in "chained", ladder-like or "twisted" form. It should not appear in yellow, deep red or bluish color. It should not have abnormal depth.

Diagnosis of Diseases through Analysis of Line of Health

A careful analysis of line of health leads to the prediction of several diseases like hepatic disorders, diseases of stomach and many other diseases of the body. While scrutinizing line of health, the medical palmist must bear the normality criteria in mind, and apply the rule, "Anything beyond normal is abnormal."

1. **Liver Disorders**

    Liver complaints are indicated by a line of health:-

    i)   Full of cuttings, breakings;

    ii)   Yellow in color;

    iii)   Chained, irregular; and

    iv)   Wavy in appearance.

Any of the four mentioned formations or appearance of line of health will indicate biliousness and liver trouble.

2. **Digestive Disorders**

Diseases of the stomach and digestive system like indigestion, impaired digestion, dyspepsia etc are indicated by a line of health if found:

        I)   Thick, ladder-like in appearance;

        ii)   Split in little pieces,

        iii)   Dots on line;

        iv)   Full of irregularities and wavy;

        v)   Crossed by deep bars; and

        vi)   Starting from line of vitality with a narrow quadrangle.

3. **Different Fevers**

Following indications on the line show fever of different types:-

I) When the line of health is very red and small spots are found, it shows a tendency in the system towards fever.

II) Brain fever is indicated by a line of health with a heavy island when joining the heart and head lines.

III) A ladder-shaped health-line shows the gastric fever.

IV) Red dots on the line of health indicate rheumatic fever.

V) When the line is red and thin in the middle, it indicates bilious fever.

4 **Other Diseases**

Besides, hepatic, gastric disorders and fevers, a number of other diseases are also indicated by the line of health which is as follows:-

I) When the line of health is feebly marked and other lines are also poor, it warns paralysis.

II) When an island is found at the commencement of the line, it denotes somnambulism.

III) When the line is red at the start especially when connected with the line of vitality, it indicates, palpitation of heart.

IV) When the line of health is touching the line of vitality it threatens severe illness.

V) When the line is broad and light, it indicates ill-health.

VI) When the hair-like lines are crossing the head and health lines, they indicate nervous troubles, headache, and troubles of stomach and liver.

VII) If a star is found in the middle of the line of health, it indicates eye-sight problem.

VIII) Serious female troubles are indicated by the line of health with a star when it is just joining the line of head, on a woman's hand.

IX) A white dot on this line shows a chronic disease.

X) A defective and poor health-line with a poor heart line indicates a defective working of heart.

XI) When an island is found near the line of health and on the line of head, it shows nose and throat troubles. When islands are found on entire line, it warns of respiratory complaints.

XII) If the line of health is red at the point where it crosses the heart-line, it denotes apoplexy.

XIII) When a star is found in the middle of the line of health, it denotes sterility.

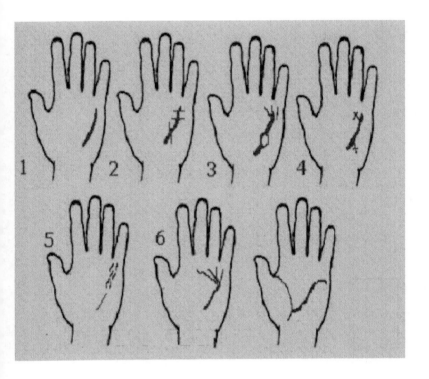

Fig. 13.2 **Different Formation of Line of Health**

CHAP: NO.14

Line of Head

1) Criteria for Normal Head-line

2) Different Formations of Head-Line

3) Diagnosis of Diseases through Analysis of Line of Head

    a. Nervous Disorders

    b. Mental Disorders

    c. Miscellaneous Disorders

Line of Head

The line of head is one of the principal diagnostic lines in the hand. It denotes a person's mental tendencies, faculties of mind, intelligence, mental control, mental health, thinking abilities, mental strain, mental attitude, degree of imagination and calculation, power of judgement, and his working condition of brain.

The line of head is associated with brain which is an organ of great complexity of structure and function. This complexity is seen in the pathological disorders of brain. In real terms, the pathology of brain is far different from the pathology of the other organs of the body. This difference is due to the fact that, brain is quite different from the other organs for its 'localization function 'i.e performance of different functions by different parts of brain.

Any defect in the normal function of brain can affect the health of entire human body. The defect may be subject to excessive concentration, abnormal mental tendencies and the imbalance in the practical and ideal views of life. The brain troubles or the disorders of the nervous system may be revealed through a careful analysis of the line of head that is closely linked with the physiology of nervous system.

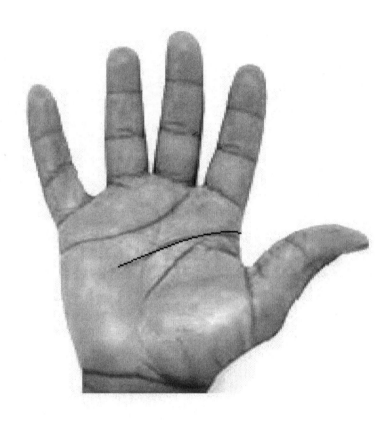

Fig. 14.1 Line of Head

1) Criteria for Normal Head-line

The line of head will be considered "normal" with the following requisites:-

    a) Normal commencement

    b) Normal course

    c) Normal termination

    d) Normal location & position

    e) Normal formation & appearance.

a) Normal Commencement

The normal commencement of the line of head is from under the mount of Jupiter, either connected or slightly separated from the line of vitality. Its commencement will be considered abnormal in the following cases:-

i) When the line of head commences from the Mount of Mars, inside the line of vitality;

11) When the gap between the line of head and line of vitality is abnormally wide;

iii) When the two lines are tightly connected for still a long course;

ix) When the line start with an island; and

x) When the line of head is simultaneously connected with the hear-line and line of vitality.

b) Normal Course

Normal course of the line of head is either straight toward percussion or gently sloping toward Mount of Moon. Its course shall be considered "abnormal" in the following cases:-

    i)   When the line of head is not connected with the line of vitality at the commencement and seems to be appearing like a bar, proceeding straight across the palm.

    Ii) When it is sloping parallel to the line of vitality like a curve; and

    iii) When the line seems to be rising toward Mount of Mercury across the line of heart.

c) Normal Termination

The normal termination of line of head is either at the second Mount of Mars forked with one prong slightly sloping toward Moon and the other resting on the Mars. Its termination shall be considered "abnormal" in the following cases:-

1)   When the line of head ends at the Mount of Moon, just reaching the wrist;

ii)   When the line is terminates at Mercury, rising upwardly;

iii)   When it terminates in the middle of the palm, under the Mount of Saturn; and

iv)   When the line terminates at the Mount of Moon with a star, undergoing"slop" toward the Mount.

d) Normal Location & Position

Normally the line of head lies not very high or low in the palm but almost in the middle of the palm i.e in the horizontal space between the first and second mounts of Mars. There should be a normal space (quadrangle) between the lines of heart and head.

e) Normal Formation & Appearance

A normal line of head appears as even, deep, straight, clear, thin, fine and free from unfavorable signs or defects. A normal line is of normal length. Its appearance and formation shall be considered "abnormal" in the following cases:-

i)   When the line of head is full of breaks or appearing to be split into little pieces;

ii)   When the line is islanded throughout its course, presenting a "chained" like formation;

iii)   When it is crisscrossed by numerous hair-like lines;

iv)   When it is appearing as "broad and shallow";

v)   When it is very red and abnormally thick and deep;

vi)   When it appears as "wavy and fading"; and

vii)   When the line of head is not free from unfavorable signs like dots, cross, circle, star, islands, grille and so on.

2) Different Formations of Head-Line

Following are the most common formations of head-lines found in the hands;

1   When the line of head is found to be separated from the line of vitality at the commencement, it denotes independence of thought and action, self-confidence, quickness in decisions and lack of caution. When the gap between the two lines is abnormally wide, it indicates over-confidence, egotism, dominance, rashness and carelessness leading to senselessness.

2   When the line of head is found to be connected with line of vitality at the commencement, it represents excess of caution, lack of self-confidence, sensitiveness, thinking abilities and power of concentration. When the connection between the two lines still goes down the hand tightly, it indicates super-sensitiveness, want of self-confidence and nervousness leading to some sort of inferiority complex, phobia or sense of vulnerability.

3   When the line of head is rising from the Mount of Mars (inside the line of vitality), it indicates extreme sensitiveness, nervousness and irritability.

4   When the line of head is straight in the first half and then slightly sloping toward Moon, it indicates a balance of imagination and reality.

5)   When the line is slightly sloping toward Moon at the center, it shows tendencies toward imaginative work and a power of imagination. When the slope is however, not "gentle" but "heavy", it is a sign of isolation from reality.

6)   When the line is forked at the termination with one prong resting on Mars and the other gently sloping toward Moon, it indicates possession of faculties of mind, both imaginative and practical.

7)   When the line is going straight to the Mars and then undergoing a gentle "curve"upward (Mercury), it indicates business talents and tendencies toward practical field of life.

8)   When the line is going straight like a bar, it indicates materialistic approach, practicability, selfishness and intellectual powers. When it is however, connected with line of vitality at the commencement, it represents an outstanding power of concentration, sympathetic attitude and an ability to think and decide.

9)   When the line ends in the middle of the hand, it indicates materialistic attitude and absence of imaginative faculties.

10) When double line of head is found, it denotes dual mentality.

3) Diagnosis of Diseases through Analysis of Line of Head

a. Nervous Disorders

The line of head when scrutinized carefully provides guidance about the subject's mental propensities, mental capacity and the nervous disorders resulting from defective working of brain and nervous system. A medical palmist can assess the mental health and predict the complications related with the nervous system analyzing the head-line applying the principle, 'Anything beyond normal is abnormal.'

i) When the line of head appears to be 'chained' or formed by a series of small islands, it indicates chronic headaches. Such a configuration also denotes weak memory.

ii) The line of head reveals the power of concentration of a subject and this power is measured in terms of the depth of this line. So when the line is abnormally deep, it indicates nervous strain resulting from excessive concentration.

iii) When the line is tightly connected with line of vitality at the start, it denotes highly sensitive nature want of self-confidence. Such a subject may be prone to inferiority complex.

iv) Insanity is warned by a head-line sloping abruptly toward the Mount of Moon.

v) When the line of head starts with an island, it indicates an inherited nervous disorder.

vi) When the line is found broken, it indicates some mental defect. If the break is serious, not mended by any small parallel line, it threatens nervous break-down.

vii) Neuralgia is indicated by a clear island on the line of head and also by a deep dent on the line.

viii) The intimacy of line of vitality and head-line for some distance at the commencement indicates brain fever.

x) A head-line rising toward line of heart indicates a tendency toward fainting fits. Other palmistic markings on hand may confirm apoplexy resulting from fainting fits.

x) When the line of head curves toward heart-line under Mount of Saturn, it indicates loss of sanity.

xi)   When light crossbars are cutting the head-line, they indicate mental confusion, depression and other brain troubles and when such deep and heavy bars terminate the line of head, they reveal some trauma of brain or injury to head.

xii)   The islands or breaks are unfavorable signs on the line of head. Whenever they appear on the line, weaken the mental-control and cause mental disbalance and loss of nervous energy.

xiii)   A line of head split into little pieces and sloping toward mount of Moon denotes a tendency toward Epilepsy.

b. Mental Disorders

1- Line of head which is tightly connected with the line of vitality at the commencement and rushes down in the same state for more than half inch, and the line appears to be very deep, it indicates a tendency toward neurotic disorders.

2- Psychotic disorders are represented by a head line full of irregularities or crossbars and terminating at mount of moon with a big slope. Sometimes there is a star or tassel at the end of head-line, which indicates a tendency toward Psychotic disorders.

c. Miscellaneous Disorders

1.   A pale and broad line of head indicates a weak memory and lack of intellectual power.

2   When a hair-like line is rushing toward mount of Venus from line of head, it indicates propensities toward mental stress. It is also considered a sign of venereal disorders, when the mount of Venus is exaggerate and red in color.

3.   When the line of head is running close to the heart line, it indicates a tendency toward Asthma or respiratory complications.

4.   When dark spots are found on the head-line, they indicate a tendency toward typhoid.

5.   When an island is found at the start of the head-line, it shows an inherited trouble.

6.   Eye-sight problems are indicated by line of head islanded or broken under mount of sun.

7.   When dots or islands are fond on the head-line under the mount of Saturn, it denotes a tendency toward deafness.

8.   A head-line termination under mount of Saturn denotes insanity.

9.   When the head-line is terminating deep into the moon and broken under Saturn, it shows a tendency toward kidney troubles.

10.   A wavy line of head indicates brain disorders.

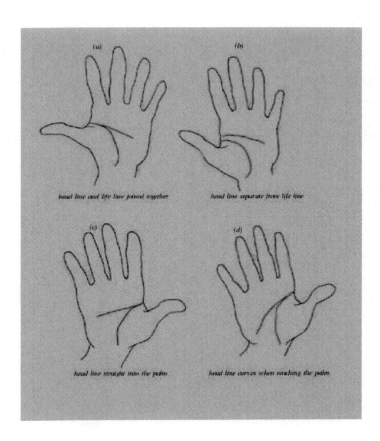

Fig. 14.2 Different Formations of Line of Head

CHAP: NO.15

Line of Heart

1)   Criteria for Normal Heart-line

2)   Different Formations of Heart-Line

3)   Diagnosis of Diseases through Analysis of Line of Heart

   a.   Cardiovascular Disorders

   b.   Personality Disorders

CHAP: NO.15

Line of Heart

Line of heart is an important diagnostic line that provides a reliable guide about the function of the heart, blood-circulation and cardio-vascular organization. It also denotes strength or weakness, kindness or hardness and warmth or coldness of heart and reveals an accurate working condition of heart. Besides cardiac disorders, a careful analysis of heart line leads to prediction of a person's emotional make-up, sex-urge and personality disorders associated with sex.

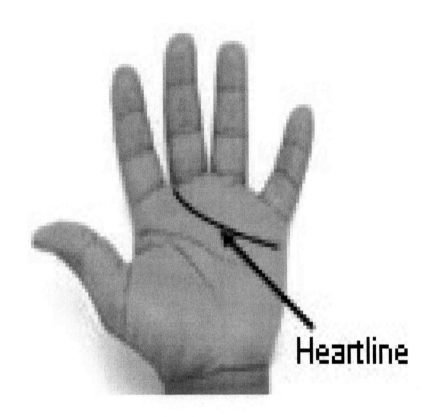

Fig. 15.1 <u>Line of Heart</u>

Criteria for Normal Heart-line

To judge an abnormality from heart-line, a medical palmist must know the normality criteria for heart-line which includes:-

i)   Normal location and position;

ii) Normal commencement and termination; and

iii) Normal formation and appearance

1)   Normal Location & Position

Normally the heart-line runs along the base (below the mounts or Mercury, Sun and Saturn) of fingers and parallel to the head-line. The line of heart must not be located at a higher or lower position in the hand.

2)   Normal Commencement & Termination

The line of heart commences from under the finger of mercury (below the mount of mercury) and runs toward the mount of Jupiter.

3)   Normal Formation & Appearance

A normal heart-line is clear, even, slightly curving or forked at its termination, and free from all defects. Its appearance and formation will be considered abnormal in the following cases:-

i)   When the heart-line is chained;

ii)   It is broken at any point;

iii) It is split intolittle pieces;

iv)   It is crisscrossed by numerous fine lines;

v)   It is broad and thick;

vi)   It is touching the head-line at the end;

vii) It is short and straight; and

viii) It is not free from unfavorable signs like dots, islands, breaks, and crossbars.

Different Formations of Line of Heart

Following are the different formations of heart-line often found in majority of hands:-

1)   When the line of heart terminates at the center of mount of Jupiter (under the finger of Jupiter) it denotes idealism in love, lack of sensuality and excess of sensitiveness.

2)   When the line of heart ends in between the finger of Saturn and Jupiter, it denotes a subject with calmer temperament in affairs of love, sound judgement, self-control and less demonstrative but deep in the feeling of love.

Diagnosis of Diseases through Analysis of Line of Heart

The line of Heart is associated with cardio-vascular system of the body. A careful scrutiny and analysis of this line predicts the action and function of the subject's heart. Heart is a vital organ. Its function is influenced by psycho-emotional episodes of the subject's life. The line of heart also indicates the pathology associated with the subject's psycho-emotional upset and sex-drive.

a) Cardio-vascular Disorders

i)   An island at any portion of heart-line denotes weak action of heart.

ii)   When the line of heart is islanded for a considerable course, it not only indicates heart trouble but also the emotional disturbance.

iii)   A wavy and thin line of heart, especially when fading, indicates poor circulation of blood, weakness of heart, lack of warmth of feelings and want of psycho-sexual energy.

iv)   When line of heart is chained throughout of its course, it denotes abnormal functioning of heart.

v)   A break in line of heart particularly under the mount of Mercury indicates a weak cardio-vascular system.

vi)   Cardiac trouble is also indicated by a big island in the line of heart.

vii)   When the line of heart is crisscrossed by several short lines, it also indicates a heart trouble.

viii)   Palpitation of heart is indicated by a dotted line of heart.

b) Personality Disorders

The line of heart gives a subject's emotional makeup, sex-drive, sensuality, sensitiveness, selfishness and attitude towards the opposite sex. A careful analysis of this line may reveal the personality disorders associated with the sex.

i)   When the line of heart is terminating at close to or almost touching the line of head under the mount of Jupiter, it denotes homosexuality. In case, when it is forked at the end with one prong touching line of head, it indicates a proclivity toward homosexuality.

ii)   A flirtatious nature is indicated by a line of heart with fine upward and downward branches arising from it.

iii)   When the line of heart terminates at the mount of Saturn under second finger it denotes sexuality, selfishness in love. When mount of Venus is red, it aggravates the subject's such attitude toward the opposite sex.

iv)   When the line of heart terminates at the center of mount of Saturn under the third finger, it denotes selfishness and absence of true affection.

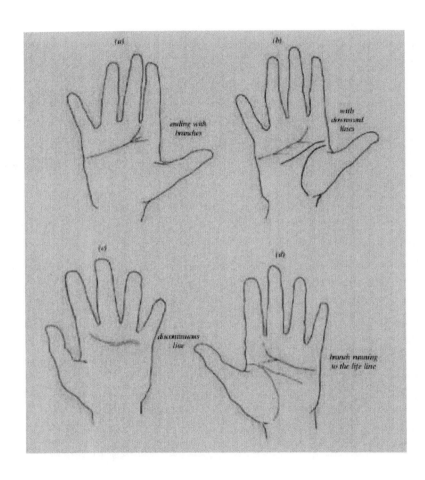

Fig. 15.2 <u>Different Formations of Line of Heart</u>

CHAP: NO: 16

Concept of 3-Hs

1- Vital organs- Brain, Heart, Liver

2- Simian Line

CHAP: NO: 16

Concept of 3-Hs

The line of Head, Heart and Health are considered as chief diagnostic lines in medical palmistry. These three lines give a concept of 3-Hs to the medical hand-analyst while reading the lines and signs of a subject's hand for the diagnosis of diseases.

1- Vital organs- Brain, Heart, Liver

The line of head mainly represents the brain and Central Nervous System (CNS) of the body. Similarly, the line of heart represents the heart and cardio-vascular system. The line of health is also called Hepatica or line of liver and represents hepatic disorders and general health problems.

From these facts about the three lines, the three vital organs- brain, heart and liver- gain importance in making a medical assessment on the basis of medical chiromancy. In order to make the concept of 3-Hs clear, it is essential to give a brief description of the vital functions which are performed by these three organs in our body.

1- Brain

Our CNS consists of the brain and the spinal cord. The brain is an extremely complex organ giving us the appreciation of sensory input. It serves as the originator and coordinator of motor activity. It acts as the repository for experience, intelligence, moral and social behavior.

Different parts of brain work together to control and moderate body activity. Cerebrum is the largest portion of the brain accounting for more than four fifths of the total brain weight. The next largest part of brain is the Cerebellum, and Brainstem, which consist of Medulla and Pons. Mid-brain is the smallest part. The more or less separate functional region that is usually described with the Cerebrum is called Dien Cephalon.

2- Heart

Heart is like a pumping machine providing the power needed for life. This life-sustaining power has, throughout time, caused an air of mystery to surround the heart. Modern technology has removed much of the mystery, but there is still an air of fascination and curiosity. The heart works tirelessly. In an average lifetime, the heart beats more than two and a half billion times, without ever pausing to rest.

3) Liver

The liver is the largest gland in the body and performs large number of tasks that impact all body systems. This is because of this fact; the hepatic disease has widespread effects on virtually all other systems of the body. Liver performs three fundamental functions:

1) Vascular functions, including formation of lymph and the hepatic phagocytic system.

2) Metabolic achievements in control of synthesis and utilization of carbohydrates, lipids and proteins.

3) Secretory and excretory functions, particularly with respect to the synthesis of secretion of bile. It is digestive function of the liver. The liver, through its biliary tract, secretes bile acids into the small intestine where they assume a critical role in the digestion and absorption of dietary lipids.

Liver disease affects people of all ages. The liver processes everything a person consumes. Among other functions, the liver cleanses the blood; regulates the supply of body fuel and manufactures many essential body proteins etc. If the liver is not properly performing its functions, the rest of the body will soon be affected by the lack of nutrients and excess waste products present in the blood. Complications arising from liver damage include fatigue, loss of appetite, lowered resistance to infections, jaundice (yellowing of the skin and eyes), and swelling of the abdomen, intestinal bleeding, brain dysfunction, and kidney failure.

In the medical Palmistry, the study of 3-Hs provides a subject's authentic profile regarding his psycho-emotional, cerebral and physiological health on the basis of which a medical palmist can make an assessment.

Brain, the power house of the body, is first affected by any disease the body suffers. This affects the blood circulation and cardio-vascular system. Heart is the center of blood circulation, which acts as pumping machine. Finally, the physiology of the body is affected as the disease gets complicated.

The signs of the disease can be analyzed by carefully scrutinizing the three lines of Head, Heart and Health.

2- Simian Line

The simian line runs across the hand replacing the heart and head line. The hands with simian lines denote a one-track mind. When such a person inclines toward some good or evil, he rushes blindly toward it. Such a person may grow as religious fanatic or a criminal. However, there is a need to look for other features and signs in the hand before reaching to a conclusion.

Simian line is considered as an abnormal sign from the diagnostic point of view. It is a sign of inner tension. It may be destructive or creative or even both. People with a simian line never really find peace. They spend their entire lives searching for an answer they never really find.

The connected lines of Heart, Head and Vitality at the commencement denote a subject with a born tendency to sticking to one cause wholeheartedly and such a person offers stubborn resistance to every hurdle or opposition in his way. This configuration also indicates proneness toward Leukemia, likely to be inherited one.

The studies have shown that simian lines may be associated with certain types of heart defects. It is also noteworthy that simian line is frequently as well observed in the hands of perfectly healthy people! In other words: a simian line has only medical value when it is observed combined with other 'medical' features in the hand.

Most of the scientific studies on the palmar lines were focussed merely on the simian line. The simian line is also indicative of Down's syndrome. However, other studies have shown that the simian line is frequently observed in other diseases and syndromes as well. The simian line combined with the dermatoglyphics on the fingertips plus the distal palmar dermatoglyphics, can be used to discriminate Down's syndrome from Edward's syndrome.

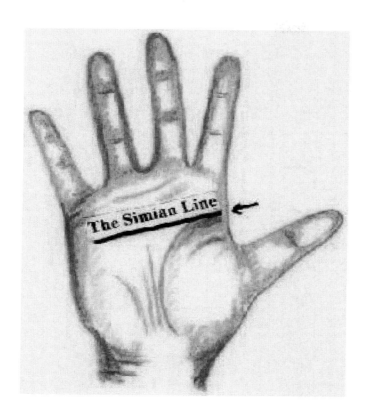

Fig. 16.1 **Simian Line**

CHAP: NO. 17

Line of Vitality

1) Criteria for Normal Vitality-line

2) Diagnosis of Diseases through Analysis of Line of Vitality

    a. Nervous Disorders

    b. Other Diseases

CHAP: NO. 17

Line of Vitality

Line of vitality or line of life is considered, an important diagnostic line in the medical palmistry which when normal in its appearance represents a robust health with good circulation of blood and a considerable reserve of vital energy. This line is located over the great palmer arch. There is a greater flow of blood through this large blood vessel which is connected with the vital organs of human body such as heart. A careful analysis of line of vitality reveals the state of a person's health, his physical constitution and complications or disorders related to the different systems of his body.

The vital energy, a person possesses is measured in terms of length of the line of vitality. A short line indicates a small and a very long line a tremendous amount of vital energy. A medical palmist should carefully scrutinize the entire course of this line, bearing in mind the criteria for a normal line of vitality.

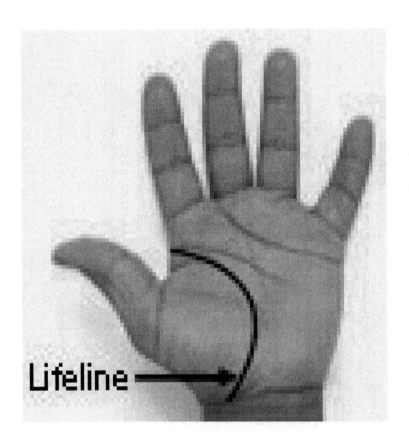

Fig. 17.1 **Line of Vitality**

1) Criteria for Normal Vitality-line

Criteria for a normal line of vitality are stated as below:-

I) Normal Location & Position

Normally, line of vitality rises under the mount of Jupiter and runs down the hand encircling the mount of Venus.

II) Normal Formation or Appearance

The line of vitality should be long, narrow, even and deep. It should be free of all sorts of irregularities or breaks. It should not appear like a chain or in a ladder-wise form. The line should not be crisscrossed by hair-like transverse lines. It should be clear and free of unfavorable signs like crossbars, spots, islands, dots etc. It should not be "forked" in its termination. It should not appear in broad and wavy form.

2) Diagnosis of Diseases through Analysis of Line of Vitality

Keeping in mind the criteria for normal appearance, location, formation and position of line of vitality in the hand, a medical palmist can diagnose the disease a person may suffer from or prone, by applying the rule, "Anything beyond normal is abnormal".

I) Nervous Disorders

Nervous disorders are indicated by a line of vitality intersected by numerous hair-like and transverse lines. When the line is found splitting into pieces (ladder-wise formation) it denotes intensity of nervousness and deficiency of nervous energy. A "chained line" also represents a nervous trouble and a delicate health.

When a fine branch is running down from line of vitality, it denotes a poor health and if the branch is spotted black it indicates nervous trouble.

Other Diseases

I)   When the line of vitality is forked at its termination or ends in a tassel, it indicates loss of vital energy.

II)   Disorder of urino-genital system is indicated by a deep crossbar terminating at mount of moon.

III)   Psychological complications are denoted by a fine line cutting the line of vitality and reaching the mount of Saturn.

I)   When the line is intersected by a fine line ending at the line of heart, it denotes some cardiac problem, the subject may prone.

V)   Feverish disposition is indicated by a line of vitality spotted red.

VI)   A break in the line shows loss of vitality, however when overlapped by a parallel line, it denotes recovery.

VII)   When the line of vitality becomes wavy and thin at any point, it denotes decline in vital force or ill-health during that period. Such a subject may be prone to pessimism and despondency.

VIII) A crowd of drooping hair-like lines is the sign of decline in vital force and ill-health.

IX)   When a bluish dot is found on the line, it indicates typhoid.

X)   A clear island at the commencement of the line indicates some inherited disease.

XI)   Disorder of respiratory system is indicated by a line of vitality that starts from the plain of mars and cuts the line of vitality terminating at the first mount of mars.

XII)   A very deep and red line denotes inflammation of walls of stomach. When the line is abnormally deep, it shows an advancing stage of paralysis.

XIII) When the line of vitality suddenly turns to the mount of moon on a woman's hand, it indicates female trouble. A square found anywhere on the line, is a sign of preservation or recovery from an illness. An island on the line denotes loss of health during that period. A black dot indicates a fatal infection.

XV) Line of mars or inner life-line gives strength to the line of vitality, when found parallel to and within it. When the line is broken at any point, the line of mars restores its vitality lost by a break.

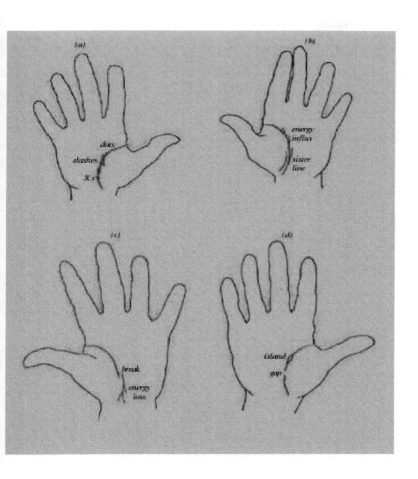

Fig. 17.2 **Different forms of Line of Vitality**

CHAP: NO: 18

Reference-Lines

1-   Line of Saturn

2.   Line of Sun

3.   Line of Mars

4.   Girdle of Venus

5.   Line of intuition

6.   Via Lasciva

7-   Three bracelets

CHAP: NO: 18

Reference-Lines

1) Line of Saturn

Normally, the line of Saturn originates from a) the Line of Life b) the middle of the palm near the wrist c) a point very near to the Line of Life: and d) the Mount of the Moon. Line of Saturn is also called the line of Fate. It may arise from the line of life, the wrist, the Mount of Venus, the line of head, or even the line of heart.

According to the traditional school of Palmistry, the line of Saturn tells all about a person's career pathway changes, independence, personal will power, and his ability to adapt to life's circumstances. Absence of this line denotes that subject's life is dictated by the circumstances. It also indicates open mindedness and freedom of decision about life.

The absence of a fate line indicates a person who lacks stability. It is also found on the hands of alcoholics and drug addicts. When line of fate is broken, it indicates a major change in a relationship or career.

When the line rises with one branch from the base of Luna, the other from Venus, The subject's destiny will sway between imagination on the one hand, while love and passion on the other.

Two fate lines are found on people who pursue two careers at the same time. If the line is tied with line of vitality at its commencement it indicates that the early portion of the subject's life will be sacrificed to the wishes of his kith and kin.

When the line of fate commences at the wrist and goes straight to the Saturn, it denotes a strong personality. It is a sign of good fortune and success.

From the Mount of Luna success is far more changeable and uncertain; fate and success will be more or less dependent on the fancy and caprice of other people. This is very often found in the case of public favorites. If the line of fate rises from the line of head and that line be well marked, then success will be won late in life after a hard struggle and through the subject's talents.

When it rises from the line of heart, it denotes success after a difficult struggle and extremely late in life. If the line of Fate is going to that of Jupiter success will be great and satisfactory.

Any break in the line is a sign of misfortune. When broken and irregular, the career will be uncertain. When there is a break in the line, it indicates loss, but if the second portion of the line being before the other leaves off, it denotes a complete change in life.

A double fate-line denotes two distinct careers. The line of fate, it has been observed, is less marked on the square and the spatulate hand, than on the conic, or the psychic.

Diagnostic value

The line of fate is not the diagnostic line but it can help the medical palmist perceive and understand the circumstances, the subject is faced with while making a medical assessment on the basis of different features of his or her hand. For example, it can give a profile of successes and failures of the subject's life and can predict the stress or tension during the critical periods of life and their effects on the health of the subject.

2) **The Line of Sun**

The line of Sun may rise from the line of life, the Mount of Luna, the Plain of Mars, the line of head, or the line of heart. All of these types should reach the Mount of Sun.

According to the traditional school, the Line of Sun is considered as the line of success. It is also called as the Apollo line. The line is deemed a sign of happiness and achievement. It is associated with a creative talent. This line indicates the success of one's efforts, whether in the acquisition of wealth, politics, a court case, travel or a love affair.

The Apollo line may commence from different points in the palm. If the Apollo line springs from the fate line it shows the point in life that the person's talents were recognized. An island on the Apollo line indicates a period where there is a loss of self esteem.

The Sun Line has been considered the sign of great luck and success in the hand by many traditional palmists. A full line of Sun starts at the base of the palm and travels up to and under the ring finger. This is a fortunate sign of creative successes or the self-confidence to make the most of inherited talents to gain possible fame in life.

It gives fame and distinction to the life when it is in accordance with the work and career given by the other lines of hand; otherwise it merely relates to a temperament that is keenly alive to the artistic, but unless the rest of the hand bears this out, the subject will have the appreciation of art without the power of expression. A star on the line of Sun indicates wealth and riches.

Rising from the line of life, with the rest of the hand artistic, it denotes that the life will be devoted to the worship of the beautiful things. With the other lines good, it promises an artistic success in artistic pursuits. Rising from the line of fate, it increases the success promised by the line of fate, and gives more distinction form whatever date it is marked - from that time things will greatly improve.

From the Mount of Luna it promises success and distinction, largely dependent upon the fancies and the help of others. In this case it is never a certain sign of success, being so influenced by fortunes of those with whom we come in contact. With a sloping line of head, however, it is more inclined to denote success in poetry, literature, and things of the purely imaginative order.

Rising upon the Plain of Mars, it promises sunshine after tears, success after difficulty. Rising from the line of head, there is no caprice of other people in connection with success, the talents of the subject alone being its factor, but until the second half of the life is reached.

Rising from the line of heart, it merely denotes a great taste for art and artistic things, and looking at it from the purely practical standpoint it denotes more distinction and influence in the world at that late date in life.

A good fate and Sun lines parallel to one another with a straight line of head is one of the greatest signs of the acquisition of wealth. The complete absence of the Line of Sun does not promise that such persons never attain fame or distinction, yet it indicates that such people no matter how hard they work find the recognition of the world hard to gain.

Diagnostic value

The line of Sun is also not the diagnostic line but a reference line. It can provide health- related information about the subject. For example, it can inform about the emotional attachments of the subject to certain goals and artistic careers in life, and for the achievement of what, the subject spends his mental and nervous energy by making efforts and struggle.

3) Line of Mars

The Line of Mars is otherwise known as the inner vital or inner life-line. It is a parallel line within the Line of Life.

It originates from the mount of Mars, runs parallel to the Line of Life towards the Mount of Venus and terminates at the wrist or the Mount of Venus.

The line of Mars denotes excess of health on all square hands to a person of this type gives a martial nature, rather a fighting disposition, and robust strength.

If it is very near the line of life or if it is very deep it indicates the extent to which a person is subject to fits of anger. If it is away from the Line of Life the person is likely to be of an equable temper. It also indicates the state of marital relations.

While it runs close to the life line it denotes the subject's fighting qualities into play. It is always an excellent sign on the hand of a soldier. When a branch shoots from this line out to the Mount of Moon, it indicates craving for excitement.

4- The Girdle of Venus

The semicircle line rising between the first and second fingers and finishing between the third and fourth is called Girdle of Venus. It may appear as 'broken or unbroken.' It denotes highly sensitive natures. Such people are moody. They are touchy over little things. It also denotes a nervous temperament, and when unbroken it indicates a tendency towards hysteria and despondency.

5- Line of Intuition

A semicircle line running from the face of the Mount of Mercury to that of the Mount of Moon is called the line of intuition. It is more often found on psychic hand.

According to the Traditional school of thought, it denotes an intuitional feeling of presentiment for others, a purely impressionable nature and strange vivid dreams.

6- The Via Lasciva

Via Lasciva is generally confounded with the line of health. It is rarely found. When running off the palm into the wrist, it gives action and force to the passion.

7- Three bracelets

Three bracelets are generally found on the wrist. When well-formed and clearly defined, they indicate strong health and a robust constitution.

When it rises into the palm like an arch, it indicates lack of potency or weakness in the relation to bearing of children.

PART IV

Palmistic Data for Various Disorders

CHAP: 19

Nervous & Mental Disorders

1- Nervous System Disorders

The nervous system is a complex, sophisticated system that regulates and coordinates body activities. It is made up of two major divisions:

- **Central nervous system** - consisting of the brain and spinal cord

- **Peripheral nervous system** - consisting of all other neural elements

Nervous disorder is a disorder of the nervous system. There are many Nervous System disorders that require clinical care by a physician. The important disorders include: Alzheimer's disease, Bell's palsy, chronic fatigue, epilepsy, convulsions, fainting, headaches, migraines, memory problems, narcolepsy, motion sickness, multiple sclerosis, paralysis, Parkinson's disease, sleep disorders, strokes, coma, vertigo.

The brain is the center that controls and regulates all voluntary and involuntary responses in the body. It consists of nerve cells that normally communicate with each other through electrical activity.

A seizure occurs when part(s) of the brain receives a burst of abnormal electrical signals that temporarily interrupt normal electrical brain function.

Amyotrophic lateral sclerosis (ALS) is a terminal neurological disorder characterized by progressive degeneration of nerve cells in the spinal cord and brain. It is one of the most devastating of the disorders that affects the function of nerves and muscles. ALS does not affect mental functioning or the senses (such as seeing or hearing), and it is not contagious.

Alzheimer's disease is a progressive, neurodegenerative disease that occurs in the brain and often results in the following:

- Impaired memory, thinking, and behavior

- Confusion

- Restlessness

- Personality and behavior changes

- Impaired judgment

- Impaired communication

- Inability to follow directions

- Language deterioration

- Impaired visuospatial skills

- Emotional apathy

Alzheimer's disease is distinguished from other forms of dementia by characteristic changes in the brain that are visible only upon microscopic examination during autopsy. Brains affected by Alzheimer's disease often show presence of the following:

- Fiber tangles within nerve cells (neurofibrillary tangles)

- Clusters of degenerating nerve endings (neuritic plaques)

Another characteristic of Alzheimer's disease is the reduced production of certain brain chemicals necessary for communication between nerve cells, especially acetylcholine, as well as norepinephrine, serotonin, and soma-tostatin.

2- Mental Disorders

`Psychiatrists have divided the mental disorders into two classes:-

A) Neurosis   B) Psychosis.

A) Neurosis

Neurotic disorders include phobias, compulsions, hysteria, hypochondria and so on.

B) Psychosis

Psychotic disorders include senile (mental disorder of old age) alcoholism, schizophrenia, depression, and so on.

Different categories of Mental disorders

a) Anxiety Disorders

Acute Stress Disorder

Panic Disorder

Agoraphobia Without History of Panic Disorder

Social Phobia

Specific Phobia (formerly Simple Phobia)

Obsessive-Compulsive Disorder

Posttraumatic Stress Disorder

Generalized Anxiety Disorder

b) Childhood Disorders

Attention-Deficit Hyperactivity Disorder

Asperger's Disorder

Autistic Disorder

Conduct Disorder

Oppositional Defiant Disorder

Separation Anxiety Disorder

Tourette's Disorder

c) Eating Disorders

Anorexia Nervosa

Bulimia Nervosa

d) Mood Disorders

Major Depressive Disorder

Bipolar Disorder (Manic Depression)

Cyclothymic Disorder

Dysthymic Disorder

e) Cognitive Disorders

Delirium

Multi-Infarct Dementia

Dementia Associated With Alcoholism

Dementia of the Alzheimer Type

Dementia

f) Personality Disorders

Paranoid Personality Disorder

Schizoid Personality Disorder

Schizotypal Personality Disorder

Antisocial Personality Disorder

Borderline Personality Disorder

Histrionic Personality Disorder

Narcissistic Personality Disorder

Avoidant Personality Disorder

Dependent Personality Disorder

Obsessive-Compulsive Personality Disorder

g) Psychotic Disorders

Schizophrenia

Delusional Disorder

Brief Psychotic Disorder

Schizophreniform Disorder

Schizoaffective Disorder

Shared Psychotic Disorder

h) Substance-Related Disorders

Alcohol Dependence

Amphetamine Dependence

Cannabis Dependence

Cocaine Dependence

Hallucinogen Dependence

Inhalant Dependence

Nicotine Dependence

Opioid Dependence

Phencyclidine Dependence

Sedative Dependence

Palmistic Data for Nervous & Mental Disorders

A- Chirognomical data

1- Following indications can be observed on the nails of a nervous patient:

I) The brittle and fluted nails indicate nervous disease.

II) When the nails are short and are very flat and sunk into flesh at the base they indicate nervous disorders.

III) White spots or dots on the nails denote nervous disease and also denote advanced stage of nervous break-down.

IV) Cross-ridges on the nails are another indication of nervousness.

V) Appearance of white dots on the nails is the first warning of delicate nerves and beginning of loss of vitality.

VI) V - Shaped nails indicate some nervous disease.

2- The third phalange (Mount of Venus) of thumb denotes not only love but sensuality, passion and sex-urge. If is short, developed and red in color, it indicates less control over passions, sensual desires and lasciviousness resulting in personality disorders.

3- If the finger of Jupiter is short (shorter than normal), it denotes inferiority complex, lack of self-confidence, dislike of responsibility, and inability to face the challenges of life. Such a subject may fall victim of frustration and despondency and may be prone to hypertension and other nervous disorders.

4- A crooked finger of Saturn denotes extreme sensitiveness and a morbid nature. Such a person may have suicidal tendencies, especially if the line of head is sloping toward luna and reaching near the wrist.

5- An excessively long finger of sun reveals a state of utopia.

6- Deviate behaviors involving inclinations toward criminal pursuits and sexual abuse are indicated by an abnormal finger of mercury when it is short and twisted. However, while making an assessment a careful analysis of mount of Venus, head-line, heart-line and thumb should be made concomitantly.

7- White hair denotes nervous diseases, especially"Shock."

8- The mount of Saturn is associated with the skeletal and nervous disorders, which are indicated by a bad mount with bad signs. When the mount is excessively developed, it denotes morbid melancholy, depression and extreme sensitiveness.

B- Chiromancy Data

1- When a network of fine lines is found in the hand, it indicates a worrying and highly nervous temperament. Such a person will have a troubled nature and may prone to anxiety, phobia, and other psychosomatic complications.

2- Wavy lines indicate insufficient flow of nervic electricity.

3- Chained lines indicate loss of nervous energy.

4- Thick lines denote lack of nervous energy.

5- Appearance of girdle of Venus in the hand denotes a nervous temperament, and when unbroken it indicates a tendency towards hysteria.

6- When line of Mars appears very deep, it indicates fits of anger.

7- The line of heart gives a subject's emotional makeup, sex-drive, sensuality, sensitiveness, selfishness and attitude towards the opposite sex. A careful analysis of this line may reveal the personality disorders associated with the sex.

v)   When the line of heart is terminating at close to or almost touching the line of head under the mount of Jupiter, it denotes homosexuality. In case, when it is forked at the end with one prong touching line of head, it indicates a proclivity toward homosexuality.

vi)   A flirtatious nature is indicated by a line of heart with fine upward and downward branches arising from it.

vii)   When the line of heart terminates at the mount of Saturn under second finger it denotes sexuality, selfishness in love. When mount of Venus is red, it aggravates the subject's such attitude toward the opposite sex.

viii) When the line of heart terminates at the center of mount of Saturn under the third finger, it denotes selfishness and absence of true affection.

8- Line of head which is tightly connected with the line of vitality at the commencement and rushes down in the same state for more than half inch, and the line appears to be very deep, it indicates a tendency toward neurotic disorders.

The line of head denotes the subject's mental propensities, mental capacity and the nervous disorders resulting from defective working of brain and nervous system.

I)   When the line of head appears to be 'chained' or formed by a series of small islands, it indicates chronic headaches. Such a configuration also denotes weak memory.

Ii)   The line of head reveals the power of concentration of a subject and this power is measured in terms of the depth of this line. So when the line is abnormally deep, it indicates nervous strain resulting from excessive concentration.

Iii)   When the line is tightly connected with line of vitality at the start, it denotes highly sensitive nature want of self-confidence. Such a subject may prone to inferiority complex.

iv)   Insanity is warned by a head-line sloping abruptly toward the Mount of Moon.

v)   When the line of head starts with an island, it indicates an inherited nervous disorder.

vi)   When the line is found broken, it indicates some mental defect. It the break is serious, not mended by any small parallel line, it threatens nervous break-down.

vii)   Neuralgia is indicated by a clear island on the line of head and also by a deep dent on the line.

viii)   The intimacy of line of vitality and head-line for some distance at the start indicates brain fever.

x)   A head-line rising toward line of heart indicates a tendency toward fainting fits. Other Palmistic markings on hand may confirm apoplexy resulting from fainting fits.

x)   When the line of head curves toward heart-line under Mount of Saturn, it indicates loss of sanity.

xi)   When light crossbars are cutting the head-line, they indicate mental confusion, depression and other brain troubles and when such deep and heavy bars terminate the line of head, they reveal some trauma of brain or injury to head.

xii)   The islands or breaks are unfavorable signs on the line of head. Whenever they appear on the line, weaken the mental-control and cause mental misbalance and loss of nervous energy.

xiii)   A line of head split into little pieces and sloping toward Mount of Moon denotes a tendency toward Epilepsy.

9- Psychotic disorders are represented by a head line full of irregularities or crossbars and terminating at mount of moon with a big slope. Sometimes there is a star or tassel at the end of head-line which indicates a tendency toward Psychotic disorders.

10- Psychological complications are denoted by a fine line cutting the line of vitality and reaching the mount of Saturn.

11- When the line of vitality becomes wavy and thin at any point, it denotes decline in vital force or ill-health during that period. Such a person may prone to pessimism and despondency.

12) Nervous disorders are indicated by a line of vitality intersected by numerous hair-like and transverse lines. When the line is found splitting into pieces (ladder-like formation), it denotes intensity of nervousness and deficiency of nervous energy.

The chained line of vitality also represents a nervous trouble and a delicate health. When a fine branch is running down from line of vitality, it denotes a poor health and if the branch is spotted black it indicates nervous trouble.

CHAP: NO. 20

Hepatic Disorders

Liver is the largest internal organ in the body. It is located in the right upper quadrant of the abdomen, immediately under the diaphragm. The liver is a complex chemical factory that works 24 hours a day. Virtually all the blood returning from the intestinal tract to the heart passes through the liver. This means everything consumed by a person that is absorbed into the bloodstream passes through the liver.

Liver is a complex but vital organ. Specifically, liver helps in:

1) Cleansing blood:

- metabolizing alcohol and other drugs and chemicals

- neutralizing and destroying poisonous substances

2) Regulating the supply of body fuel:

- producing, storing and supplying quick energy (glucose) to keep the mind alert and the body active

- producing, storing and exporting fat

3) Manufacturing many essential body proteins involved in:

- transporting substances in the blood

- clotting of blood

- providing resistance to infection

4) Producing bile which eliminates toxic substances from the body and aids digestion

5) Regulating the balance of many hormones:

- sex hormones

- thyroid hormones

- cortisone and other adrenal hormones

6) Regulating body cholesterol by producing it, excreting it, and converting it to other essential substances.

7) Regulating the supply of essential vitamins and minerals such as iron and copper. Experimentally, it has been proved that excretion of more than 80% hepatic parenchyma is related to the normal function of liver. It has an enormous reserve capacity. When depletion of the functional reserve happens, it causes two common hepatic disorders!

1. Jaundice   2. Liver failure.

1. **Jaundice**

It is a hepatic disorder in which skin becomes yellowish in color. This yellow discoloration of skin is produced by accumulation of bilirubin in the tissues.

Jaundice is caused by the disturbance in equilibrium between the production and disposal of bilirubin which occurs due to its excessive production or its inhibition of outflow. The intensity of the disease depends on the rate of diffusion of bilirubin from plasma into interstitial fluid which results in its accumulation in the tissues. Most frequent causes of Jaundice in adults are viral hepatitis, drug reactions, and extra-hepatic biliary obstruction.

2.   Liver Failure

Numerous hepatic diseases like erosion of functional reserve of liver or a severe infection ultimately result in liver failure.

There are over 100 known liver diseases. The most common ones such as gallstones, viral hepatitis, cirrhosis, cancer of the liver and some children's liver diseases.

Palmistic Data for Hepatic Disorders

1- When the palm is yellowish or blue in color, it indicates biloiusness.

2- Bilousness is also indicated by the mount of Mercury crisscrossed by many fine lines.

3. When lines appear as yellow in color, the subject may be prone to hepatic disorders.

4. Liver complaints are indicated by a line of health:-

       i)   Full of cuttings, breakings;

       ii)   Yellow in color;

       iii)   Chained, irregular; and

       iv)   Wavy in appearance.

Any of the four mentioned formations or appearance of line of health will indicate biliousness and liver trouble.

5-   When the line of health is red and thin in the middle, it indicates bilious fever.

CHAP: NO.21

Disorders of Immunity

The various disorders of immunity may be classed as under:

1.   Auto-immune diseases

2.   Immuno-deficiency diseases.

I)   AUTO-IMMUNE DISEASE

Self-tolerance is necessary for our tissues to live harmoniously with an army of lymphocytes (White blood cells). Breakdown of one or more of the mechanisms of self-tolerance can unleash an immunologic attack on tissues that lead to the development of auto-immune diseases.

Most important auto-immune diseases include Rheumatoid arthritis, systematic sclerosis, polymyositis-dermatomyostis and polyarteritis Nodosa.

a)   Rheumatoid Arthritis:

This is auto-immune disease which is caused by persistent inflammation resulting from immunologic processes taking place in Joints. It affects principally the small joints of hands and feet, ankles, wrists, elbows and shoulders.

b)   Systemic Sclerosis:

This is an autoimmune disease which is characterized by inflammatory changes in many organs of the body. The most prominent changes are found in skin, lungs, heart, kidney and gastrointestinal tract.

c)   Polymyositis-dermatomyositis:

This is a disease characterized by inflammation of muscles and skin rash.

d)   Polyarteritis Nodosa:

This is an autoimmune disease characterized by inflammation of arteries.

II)   Immuno Deficiency Diseases

Some of the Immuno deficiency diseases are as described below:

a) **Thymic Hypoplasia:**

This is a disease caused by deficiency of thymus which makes the infants vulnerable to viral, fungal and bacterial infections.

b) **AIDS:**

Acquired Immuno deficiency syndrome (AIDS) is deadly lethal disease which is caused by Human Immuno deficiency virus (HIV). The Aids virus transmits through sexual contact, Intravenous drug administration by contaminated needles, and transmission through blood administration and from infected mother to newborn babies. AIDS destroys the whole immune system of the body and patient is vulnerable to attack of any kind of infection.

Palmistic Data for Immunity Disorders

1- Rheumatoid arthritis is indicated by nails with longitudinal ridges, especially when splitting at the ends.

2- The mount of Saturn with grill or with many short vertical lines also denotes proneness to arthritis.

3- The phalanges of fingers appear as deformed in the hands of arthritis patient.

4- When a line with islands is running from line of vitality toward mount of Saturn, it also indicates proneness to arthritis.

CHAP: NO. 22

Genetic Disorders

Most important genetic disorders are as under:

I) **Diabetes Mellitus**

Diabetes mellitus is a genetic disease which affects the carbohydrate, fate and protein metabolism. This disease is characterized by a deficient insulin secretory response. Insulin is a major Harmon which is synthesized by the beta cells of pancreas. It is necessary for transport of glucose, protein synthesis, glycogen formation and for conversion of glucose to triglycerides. All the diabetics have absolute lack of insulin and thus they suffer from an inability to utilize glucose adequately resulting in an accumulation of glucose in the blood.

II) **Gout**

Gout is a genetic disorder of uric acid metabolism which is characterized by the elevation of the level of serum uric Acid due to its over-production, or reduced excretion. A plasma urate value above 7-mg/100ml is considered "elevated."

The progressive accumulation of urates and thus recurrent attacks of inflammation lead to chronic arthritis. Then the urates deposit in and around the joints. These deposits create mass urates which is morphologically known as Tophus. As tophi develop in joints, the cartilage and bone are eroded and thus a progressive destruction of joint continues. So Gout in fact, is a persistent disabling joint disease. Tophi-- the morphologic hallmark of gout may develop in particular ligaments, connective tissues, and the ear-lobes. Sometimes, they appear on the palm of the hand or skin of the fingertips and less frequently, they appear in kidneys.

Palmistic Data for Genetic Disorders

1- A distorted finger of mercury signifies trickery and a devilish mentality. Such a finger sometimes indicates a genetic disorder of thyroid secretion

2- A clear island at the commencement of the line indicates some inherited disease.

3- Diabetes is indicated by a deep cross at the mount of moon. Sometimes the mount is crisscrossed by numerous fine lines.

4- When a star on the lower part of mount of moon is found and it sends off a fine line running toward and crossing the line of vitality, this sign is also indicative of diabetes.

CHAP.NO: 23

Gastro-Intestinal Disorders

Most common Gastro-intestinal disorders are as follows:-

I)   **Gastritis**

Inflammation of the walls of stomach is generally refereed to gastritis. It may be either erosive or non-erosive. An erosive gastritis is always marked by a layering of the gastric lining with partially digested blood and by prominent inflammatory mucosal infiltrate. A non-erosive gastritis is characterized by mucosal chronic inflammatory changes.

Though the two categories of Gastritis (erosive & non-erosive) are different and unrelated but both damage the gastric mucosa.

II)   **Peptic ulcers**

Peptic ulcers are actually the mucosal holes in any portion of Gastro-intestinal tract which are the consequences of aggressive action of acid-pepsin secretion and weakened defenses of the gastrointestinal mucosa.

When peptic ulcers are located in duodenum, they are called as duodenal ulcers, and when in the stomach, they are named as gastric ulcers.

III)   **Diarrhea**

The Diarrhea is a common intestinal disorder which is principally marked by an increase in stool water leading to an increase in the number of bowel movements. It results from excessive intestinal mucosal secretion, which overwhelms the absorptive capacity of the colon. A diarrheal disease is caused by enteric pathogens.

IV)   **Cholera**

It is a diahrreal disease caused by bacterium-- vibro cholera.

V)   **Bacillary Dysentery**

It is another diarrheal disease which is caused by a bacterium--shigella. The disease is characterized by lower abdominal pain and the passage of watery stools containing pus.

VI)   Typhoid Fever

Typhoid fever is also caused by a bacterium-- salmonella typhi and is characterized as prolonged illness. The infection begins with a fever that progressively mounts each day.

Despite the high fever, the slow pulse-rate, abdominal pain and constipation alternating with diarrhea are other features of typhoid.

VII) Colitis

The inflammation of colon, a part of large intestine, is called colitis. It may be either pseudomembranous when caused by a bacterium-clostridium difficile or amebic when caused by a protozoan--Entamoeba histolytica. The disease is characterized by abdominal cramps, and diarrhea.

VIII) Appendicitis

Appendicitis is the most common gastrointestinal disease which is referred to an inflammation of appendix. The condition is characterized by discomfort, nausea, vomiting and distended appendix.

Palmistic Data for Gastro-Intestinal Disorders

1- When the palm of the hand is yellowish in color, it indicates intestinal disorders like dyspepsia, and defect in parastalysis.

2- The bending nail phalange of finger of Saturn toward the finger of sun indicates some intestinal disorders. However before making an assessment, some other signs of intestinal disorder from the hand must be confirmed.

3- The nails with longitudinal ridges indicate colitis.

4- A ladder-shaped health-line shows the gastric fever.

5- Diseases of the stomach and digestive system like indigestion, impaired digestion, dyspepsia etc are indicated by a line of health if found:

        i)   Thick, ladder-like in appearance;

       ii)   Split in little pieces,

      iii)   Dots on line;

      iv)   Full of irregularities and wavy;

v)   Crossed by deep bars; and

vi)   Starting from line of vitality with a narrow quadrangle.

6. When the lines are dark in color, the subject may be prone to gastritis.

7. A ladder-shaped health-line shows the gastric fever.

8- When a bluish dot is found on the line of vitality, it indicates typhoid.

9- A very deep and red line of vitality denotes gastritis.

CHAP: NO.24

Cardiovascular Disorders

Following are the most common heart diseases or cardiac disorders:

I)   Coronary heart disease

It is a cardiac disorder which results from an imbalance between myocardial need for oxygen and its supply. This imbalance is created when the coronary arteries are narrowed due to Atherosclerosis, and thus sufficient amount of blood does not flow through them.

II)   Hypertensive Heart Disease

This disease is characterized by thickening of left ventricle and an increase in the weight of heart. In fact, a prolonged hypertension badly affects the working of heart and leads to this disease.

III)   Rheumatic Fever

Rheumatic fever is a systemic and inflammatory disease in which heart; blood vessels, skin and the joints are largely affected. When heart is severely involved, the disease is called Rheumatic heart disease.

IV)   Pericarditis

The inflammation of Pericardium (the membrane enclosing heart) is known as Pericarditis. Generally it is caused by some microbiologic infections.

V)   Congestive Heart Failure

It is caused by coronary heart disease and hypertension. The disease is characterized by the inability of the cardiac output to keep pace with veinous return. This eventually results in blood damming back into the veinous system which leads to diminished filling of arterial pathways.

The heart becomes dilated and the additional blood volume stresses the heart by producing congestion. One side of heart begins to fail which ultimately results in total heart failure.

B- Vascular Disorders

Vascular system disorders may be divided into two groups:

I) Arterial Diseases

Common arterial diseases are:

a) Arteriosclerosis:

This is a vascular disorder causing thickening and inelasticity of arteries. In fact, it is a disease of small arteries and arterioles mostly associated with hypertension and diabetes mellitus.

b) Atherosclerosis:

This disease is characterized by the formation of initial fibro-fatty lesions which cause narrowing of vascular lumen. The centers of these lesions contain lipid-rich debris consisting of cholesterol.

II) Venous Disorders

Common venous disorders are as under:-

a) Varicose veins:

Varicose veins are abnormally dilated and induce a great deal of discomfort. The common cause of this disorder is increased intraluminal pressure. In this condition, the affected veins are elongated and irregularly dilated.

b) Phlebothrombosis:

This is condition characterized by thrombus formation most often within deep veins of lower extremities, particularly the macular veins of the calf.

Phlebothrombosis is commonly associated with cardiac failure, prolonged bed rest, post-operative states and any form of severe trauma, particularly extensive burns.

Palmistic Data for Cardiovascular Disorders

1- A crooked finger of sun is a sign of heart disease.

2- The following indications and symptoms of weak heart and poor circulation of blood can be observed on the nails:

I) Blueness at the base of any nail indicates a weak heart and poor circulation of blood.

II) When blueness is observed at the base of small tapering nails with the end quite square, and tapering towards the base, it means pronounced heart trouble.

III) At the base of the nail there is a curved white portion, which is called as moon.

a) Small moons indicator weak action of heart and poor circulation of blood.

b) Large moons indicate rapid circulation of blood and a strong action of heart.

c) Very large of the moons on the nails denote much pressure on the heart.

d) The nails without moons show an advanced stage of the disease.

IV) Conical nails indicate poor physical health and blood circulatory system.

V) If long nails are bluish in color and are wider at the top, the blood circulation will be the result.

VI) If blueness is found on the nails at the age of 12 to 14 years, it would be temporary obstruction of blood circulation and would not be taken as serious one. But if blueness is found at the age of 18 to 42 years it indicates serious trouble. When again found at the age of 43 to 47 it denotes a difficulty of probably short duration.

VII) Short and pale nails indicate anemia, and physical weakness.

3)   When the line of vitality is intersected by a fine line ending at the line of heart, it denotes some cardiac problem, the subject may be prone.

4)   A defective and poor health-line with a poor heart line indicates a defective working of heart.

5)   The line of heart indicates the following cardio vascular disorders:-

i)   An island at any portion of heart-line denotes weak action of heart.

ii)   When the line of heart is islanded for a considerable course, it not only indicates heart trouble but also the emotional disturbance in the subject.

iii) A wavy and thin line of heart, especially when fading, indicates poor circulation of blood, weakness of heart, lack of warmth of feelings and want of psycho-sexual energy.

iv) When line of heart is chained throughout of its course, it denotes abnormal functioning of heart.

v) A break in line of heart particularly under the mount of Mercury indicates a weak cardio-vascular system.

vi) Cardiac trouble is also indicated by a big island in the line of heart.

vii) When the line of heart is crisscrossed by several short lines, it also indicates a heart trouble.

viii) Palpitation of heart is indicated by a dotted line of heart.

6- Red dots on the line of health indicates rheumatic fever.

CHAP: NO.25

Cell Disorders

Blood cell disorders may be classed as:

I)   Red cell disorders   II)   White cell disorders

I)   **Red Cell Disorders**

The most common red cell disorders are as follows:-

a)   **Anemia**

Anemia is considered as a reduction (below normal levels) of hemoglobin concentration. Hemoglobin is an iron pigment of red color which is necessary for transport of oxygen to the tissues of the body. So the disease results in an impaired delivery of oxygen to the tissues.

b)   **Sickle Cell Disease**

It is a hereditary disorder of red cells which is characterized by the presence of structurally abnormal hemoglobin. The shape of red cells becomes elongated and anemia is worsened in the sickle cell disease.

c)   **Malaria**

Malaria is caused by malarial parasite- plasmodium- which is transmitted to man by the bite of a female anopheles mosquito. Disease is characterized by a feeling of cold & shivering, high fever and profuse sweats. The parasites destroy large number of red cells and cause anemia.

d)   **Erythrocytosis**

This is a disease which is characterized by an increase in hemoglobin (red cell mass) level and a decrease in plasma level. It is caused by dehydration that may be associated with prolonged vomiting or diarrhea.

II) White Cell Disorders

Following are the important white cell disorders:-

a) Lymphomas

Lymphoid tissue contains lymphocytes and histiocytes. When there is an accumulation of cells native to lymphoid tissue, this is referred to a cancer of lymphoid tissue or lymphomas.

b) Leukemia

It is commonly known as blood cancer, which is characterized by diffuse replacement of the bone marrow by neoplastic cells. The leukemic cells spill over in blood in large number. They may also spread through out the body.

c) Hemophilia

It is a hereditary disorder of platelets which results in deficiency of blood clotting factor.

Palmistic Data for Cell Disorders

1- When the color of the palm is white, it indicates lack of blood supply and lack of red blood cells (RBCs) in the blood.

2- Anemia is indicated by the short and colorless nails.

3 - An excessively pale palm also denotes anemia.

4- Pale lines indicate lack of vitality, poor circulation of blood and deficiency of red blood cells in the blood.

5- The presence of simian line indicates a risk of leukemia.

6- A broken line of health, particularly when it appears as very thin line, indicates Malaria.

7- The connected lines of Heart, Head and Vitality at the commencement indicates proneness toward Leukemia, likely to be inherited one.

8- The risk of Malaria is also indicated by bluish or black dots on the lines of Heart and Head.

CHAP: NO.26

Venereal &Urino-genital Disorders

The Syphilis and Gonorrhea are the important and most serious venereal disorders, which are spread by sexual contact. The genital tract is attacked in these disorders.

The disorders of the Urino-genital tract include Irregularities of menstruation, displacement of the uterus, sexual weakness.

Menstruation is uterine bleeding which occurs at intervals of 24 to 32 days in the normal woman during the reproductive years. Ovulation and the resulting production of estrogen and progesterone hormones results in bleeding, when pregnancy does not occur. Irregularities of menstruation may indicate disease or deficiency states or emotional disturbance or hormonal imbalance.

Excessive bleeding during the normal time is called hypermenorrohea. Prolonged bleeding is called menorrhagia. Painful menstruation or dysmenorrhea is characterized by cramps in the lower abdomen and discomfort.

Metrorrhagia means irregular flow at times other than the normal menstrual period. In olygomenorrhea there is scanty discharge.

Palmistic Data for Venereal & Urino-genital Disorders

1- The finger of mercury is believed to be connected with urino- genital system. If the third phalange of this finger is thick and a deep vertical line is cutting the second phalange, it is a sign of urino-genital disorder.

2- Delicate and narrow nails are an indication of a delicate constitution

3- Long, brittle and convex nails are indicative of venereal disorders.

4- Three bracelets, when poorly formed and not clearly defined, they indicate sexual weakness. When it rises into the palm like an arch, it indicates lack of potency or weakness in the relation to bearing of children.

5- Disorder of Urino-genital system is indicated by the line of vitality with a deep crossbar terminating at mount of moon.

6- When the line of Vitality suddenly turns to the mount of moon on a woman's hand, it indicates female trouble.

7-   When a star is found in the middle of the line of health, it denotes sterility.

8-   Serious female troubles are indicated by the line of health with a star when it is just joining the line of head, on a woman's hand.

9-   Female troubles are also indicated by mount of Venus if it is undeveloped and with numerous vertical lines.

10-   The much-lined mounts of Saturn and Moon also denote female troubles.

11-   When a star is found under the finger of Saturn with a triple broken girdle of Venus, it indicates high risk of Syphilis and Gonorrhea.

12-   When the line of vitality is found 'broken' in both hands, it also denotes proneness to venereal diseases.

13- When a hair-like line is rushing toward mount of Venus from line of head, it indicates venereal disorders particularly when the mount of Venus is exaggerate and red in color.

14- When the mount of Venus is found as depressed or deficient, it indicates coldness of heart and feelings, deficient sex-urge, poor health and cold nature.

CHAP: 27

Throat & Respiratory Disorders

The respiratory system consists of the nose, pharynx, larynx, trachea, bronchi and lungs. The upper respiratory tract includes the nose, nasal cavity, ethmoidal air cells, frontal sinuses, maxillary sinus, larynx, and trachea. And the lower respiratory tract includes the lungs, bronchi and alveoli.

The lungs are a pair of cone-shaped organs made up of spongy, pinkish-gray tissue. They take up most of the space in the chest. They take in oxygen, which cells need to live and carry out their normal functions. The lungs also get rid of carbon dioxide, a waste product of the body's cells.

Throat & Respiratory Disorders include the upper Respiratory Infections and Lung Disorders.

Upper Respiratory Infections

- Common Cold

- Influenza

- Pharyngitis / Tonsillitis

- Sinusitis

Lung Disorders

- Chronic Obstructive Pulmonary Disease (COPD)

- Asthma

- Chronic Bronchitis

- Pulmonary Emphysema

- Acute Bronchitis

- Cystic Fibrosis

- Interstitial Lung Diseases / Pulmonary Fibrosis

- Occupational Lung Diseases

- Pneumonia

- Primary Pulmonary Hypertension

- Pulmonary Embolism

- Pulmonary Sarcoidosis

- Tuberculosis

- Lung Cancer

- Sleep Problems

- Insomnia

Palmistic Data for Respiratory Disorders

1- Nails denote the following respiratory disorders:-

) - Curved nails indicate delicacy of bronchial tubes and weakness of lungs.

II) - Clubbed nails are indicative of tuberculosis and lung disease.

III)   Very long nailed persons may be prone to suffer from chest and lung disease.

2- When the line of head is running close to the heart line, it indicates a tendency toward Asthma or respiratory complications.

3- Disorder of respiratory system is indicated by a line of Vitality that starts from the plain of mars and cuts the line of vitality terminating at the first mount of mars.

4- When an island is found near the line of health and on the line of head, it shows nose and throat troubles.   When islands are found on entire line, it warns of respiratory complaints.

CHAP: 28

Renal or Urologic Disorders

Any disorder of the kidneys or the urinary tract is called renal or urologic disorder. Kidney disease is classified as any disease or disorder that affects the function of the kidneys.

Renal or urologic disorders may include:

- Acute kidney failure
- Acute nephritic syndrome
- Analgesic nephropathy
- Atheroembolic renal disease
- Chronic kidney failure
- Chronic nephritis
- Congenital nephrotic syndrome
- End-stage renal disease
- Goodpasture's syndrome
- IgM mesangial proliferative glomerulonephritis
- Interstitial nephritis
- Kidney cancer
- Kidney damage
- Kidney infection
- Kidney injury
- Kidney stones

- Lupus nephritis

- Membranoproliferative GN I

- Membranoproliferative GN II

- Membranous nephropathy

- Minimal change disease

- Necrotizing glomerulonephritis

- Nephroblastoma

- Nephrocalcinosis

- Nephrogenic diabetes insipidus

- Nephropathy - IgA

- Nephrosis (nephrotic syndrome)

- Polycystic kidney disease

- Post-streptococcal GN

- Reflux nephropathy

- Renal artery embolism

- Renal artery stenosis

- Renal disorders

- Renal papillary necrosis

- Renal tubular acidosis type I

- Renal tubular acidosis type II

- Renal underperfusion

- Renal vein thrombosis

Palmistic Data for Renal Disorders

1- When the nail phalange of the finger of Mercury appears to be bending inward over palm, it reveals renal disorders.

2- When the head-line is terminating deep into the moon and broken under Saturn, it shows a tendency toward kidney troubles.

3- Much –lined mount of Moon (lower part) also indicates renal disorders.

4- If a line runs from mount of Moon toward line of vitality and is forked at the end, it also denotes kidney ailments.

CHAP: 29

Palmistic Data for Miscellaneous Disorders

1- Paralysis

When the line of health is feebly marked and other lines are also poor, it warns paralysis. other signs include short and triangular nails, much-lined and an elevated mount of Saturn and a star at the end of line of vitality.

2- Headaches

A chained and broken head-line and an irregular but red line of health indicate chronic headaches.

3- Piles

Hemorrhoids or Piles is indicated by a much-lined and elevated mount of Saturn. A dotted line of vitality sending off a fine branch toward upper mount of Mars that terminates in a star also indicates high risk of piles.

4- Eye problems

Eye-sight problems are indicated by line of head islanded or broken under mount of sun. If a star is found in the middle of the line of health, it also indicates eye-sight problem. Other signs include much-lined mount of sun and defective line of sun.

5- Deafness

When dots are found on the head-line under the mount of Saturn, it denotes a tendency toward deafness.

6- Insanity

A head-line termination under mount of Saturn denotes insanity. If the head-line is sloping down and terminating at mount of Moon with a star also denotes insanity. Other signs include an elevated mount of Moon and a head-line crisscrossed by many fine lines.

7- Blood pressure

When the lines of hand appear to be red in color, the subject may be prone to high blood pressure.

8- Skin diseases

The skin diseases are indicated by a hand with short nails, chained line of heart and ladder-like appearance of the line of health.

9- Suicide

A very long finger of Saturn will show morbid desires, melancholy and a pessimistic behavior. Such a person may prone to retardation and pessimism which may lead him to isolation from the world or to suicide ultimately (if other unfavorable signs are also present in hand). When the finger of Saturn is found to be 'crooked', it denotes extreme sensitiveness and a morbid nature. Such a person may have tendencies toward suicide especially if the line of head is sloping toward luna and reaching near the wrist.

10- Drug addiction

The drug or narcotics addiction is indicated by a hand with an abnormal thumb, elongated mount of Moon and a weak line of head.

CHAP: NO. 30

Case Study

1- Hand of A Drug Addict

This is the hand print of a drug addict; I met with in Quetta Pakistan. Haji Muhammed was an Afghan refugee, who lost his family and everything in war-torn Afghanistan. He was married and father of 8 children. He was a peasant by profession. The war in Afghanistan brought destruction in his life and made him a refugee. He was in deep woe and frustration. An analysis of his hand indicates his mental disturbance and a life replete with trial and tribulation.

A break in line of head shows that he had lost nervous energy and power of survival and finally he took refuge in narcotics. Ultimately, he became a narcotics addict. An important feature of the hand is the simian line. It has been observed that, a person with a simian line never really finds peace. He spends his entire life searching for an answer he never really finds.

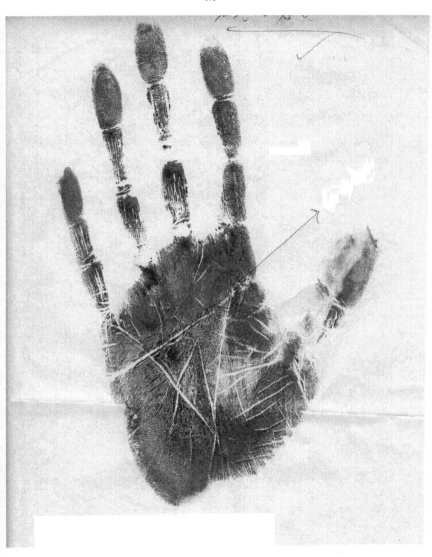

Fig. 30.1 Hand **of a drug addict**

2- Hand of a Cancer Patient

I met with Nazo Bibi, a cancer patient, in Quetta, Pakistan. She was 45 years old. She was suffering from thigh cancer. She died in June 1999.

The hand of Nazo shows a network of lines. The head-line is crisscrossed by several small lines. The several bars seem to be crossing the line of vitality from mount of Venus. There are also two islands on the line of health. All these signs and markings on the palm indicate a poor health and loss of hope.

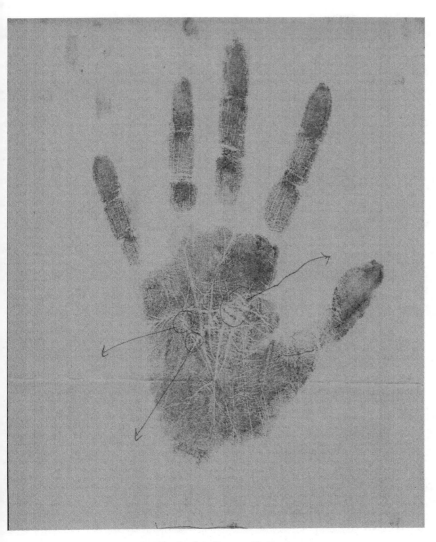

Fig. 30.2 **Hand of A Cancer Patient**

Selected Bibliography

1- P.G Zimbardo, A.L Weber, *psychology*, second edition, 1997, USA

2- S. L Robbins, V. Kumar, *Basic Pathology*, 4th Edition, NBF 1st reprint 1989.

3- Marten Steinbach, *Medical Palmistry*, 1976, USA.

4- L. R. Chawdhary, *A handbook of Palmistry*, 1987, India

5- Cheiro, *Cheiro's Guide to the Hand*, 9th edition, 1985, printed in India

<u>6-</u> **Hand Anatomy:** *Bradon J Wilhelmi*, MD, Professor and Endowed Leonard J Weiner, MD, Chair of Plastic Surgery, Residency Program Director, University of Louisville School of Medicine(http://emedicine.medscape.com/article/1285060-overview)

<u>Web References</u>

www.handresearch.com

www.liver.ca

www.bigeye.com

www.mentalhealth.com
www.dermatoglyphics.com

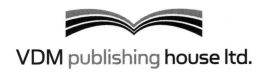
 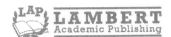 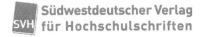

Printed in Great Britain
by Amazon

24586984R00106